Current Fracture Care

Edited by John T. Riehl
and Jan P. Szatkowski

Published in London, United Kingdom

Current Fracture Care
http://dx.doi.org/10.5772/intechopen.104181
Edited by John T. Riehl and Jan P. Szatkowski

Contributors
Ali Zamanian, Alvaro Zamorano, Grayson A. Domingue, Jan P. Szatkowski, John Thomas Riehl, Louise M. Richardson, Luis Bahamonde, Martin D. Richardson, McKenna W. Box, Mostafa Shahrezaei, Neil J. Werthmann, Nikolaos Laliotis

First published in London, United Kingdom, 2024 by IntechOpen
IntechOpen is the global imprint of INTECHOPEN LIMITED, registered in England and Wales, registration number: 11086078, 167-169 Great Portland Street, London, W1W 5PF, United Kingdom

British Library Cataloguing-in-Publication Data
A catalogue record for this book is available from the British Library

Additional hard and PDF copies can be obtained from orders@intechopen.com

Current Fracture Care
Edited by John T. Riehl and Jan P. Szatkowski
p. cm.
Print ISBN 978-1-80356-755-6
Online ISBN 978-1-80356-756-3
eBook (PDF) ISBN 978-1-80356-757-0

For EU product safety concerns:
IN TECH d.o.o., Prolaz Marije Krucifikse Kozulić 3, 51000 Rijeka, Croatia,
info@intechopen.com or visit our website at intechopen.com.

Meet the editors

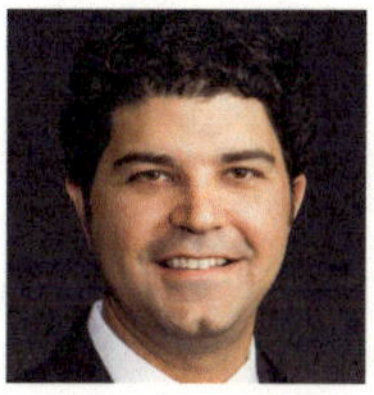

Dr. John Riehl attended California Lutheran University College in Southern California where he majored in biochemistry and molecular biology, graduating with honors and receiving a Bachelor of Science degree. He attended Temple University School of Medicine, PA, USA, where he encountered a hands-on clinical experience that helped to instill within him the caring and compassionate approach that he continues to bring to his patients every day. Dr. Riehl performed his orthopaedic surgery residency in rural Pennsylvania at Geisinger Medical Center. It was at Geisinger where Dr. Riehl learned to approach orthopaedic surgery in a comprehensive manner and to bring the best available innovation to his patients. Dr. Riehl became heavily involved in orthopedic research during his residency as well, where he published eleven research papers and three textbook chapters on topics ranging from foot disorders to multiligamentous knee injuries (Dr. Riehl has continued his quest to further orthopaedic knowledge and innovation since residency. For a full list of his publications visit https://www.johnriehl.com/publications/). Dr. Riehl received subspecialty training in fracture care at Orlando Regional Medical Center, a high-volume trauma center in Orlando, Florida. It was there that Dr. Riehl cultivated his expertise in pelvic and acetabular surgery and all aspects of fracture care. After his fellowship, Dr. Riehl went into practice at the University of Louisville, KY, USA, where he was an assistant professor of orthopaedic surgery and served as the associate residency program director. Dr. Riehl received the prestigious award of the Best Faculty Educator of the residents two years in a row while at the University of Louisville. From Louisville, Dr. Riehl brought his medical practice to Pensacola, FL where he served the Gulf Coast for nearly 7 years. There, Dr. Riehl developed and implemented protocols across specialty lines to improve patient care and continued to publish research. During this time, Dr. Riehl also traveled part-time and held the position of director of orthopaedic trauma at a trauma center in eastern Kentucky, bringing expert orthopaedic care to an underserved area. Additionally, he has held positions for many years on the editorial board of an orthopaedic journal, a popular orthopaedic website, and the review board of two others. Dr. Riehl remains active in academics, working with residents and medical students in research endeavors. Dr. Riehl is currently the residency program director for the Medical City UNT/TCU Orthopaedic Surgical Residency in Denton, Texas, which operates throughout the Dallas/Fort Worth area. Dr. Riehl has committed his career to serving the communities where he has practiced while providing the highest quality of care, always putting the patient first. Dr. Riehl currently lives and practices in the Dallas/Fort Worth area and continues his dedication to the field of orthopaedic surgery. In addition to the current text, Dr. Riehl has authored a book describing diet and exercise (*Intelligent Carb*) and has authored and edited a book about tibial plateau fractures (*Tibial Plateau Fractures*).

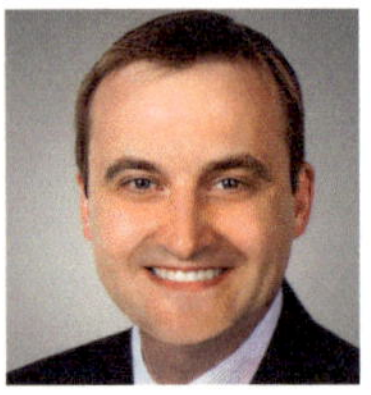

Dr. Jan Szatkowski is a dual fellowship-trained orthopedic trauma and foot and ankle surgeon at Indiana University, USA, where he serves as Director of Orthopaedic Trauma and Director of Foot and Ankle. His expertise is in managing the most complex orthopedic cases to prevent or reduce permanent disability. Dr. Szatkowski offers comprehensive care for a wide range of orthopedic conditions, including simple and complex fractures, post-traumatic arthritis, revision surgery, and joint replacement surgery (hip and ankle). Dr. Szatkowski's commitment to advancing orthopedic care is evident in his active involvement in the research and development of new medical technologies. He has co-authored numerous articles in scientific journals, contributing valuable knowledge to the field. His research focuses on innovations that promise to enhance orthopaedic treatment and patient outcomes. Beyond his technical expertise, Dr. Szatkowski is known for his patient-centered approach to care. He believes in open, honest communication and treats each patient as a whole, considering all aspects of their health and well-being. This holistic perspective ensures that each patient receives the most effective treatment tailored to their unique situation. Dr. Szatkowski's academic background includes an undergraduate degree from Duke University and a medical degree from the University of Chicago's Pritzker School of Medicine. He completed his residency at the Mayo Clinic, MN, USA, and pursued fellowships in orthopaedic trauma and foot and ankle surgery at the Campbell Clinic-University of Tennessee, USA. He is certified by the American Board of Orthopaedic Surgery. Dr. Szatkowski's roles as Director of Orthopaedic Trauma and Director of Foot and Ankle at Indiana University highlight his leadership within the field and his dedication to improving the lives of his patients through exceptional care and innovative treatment solutions. Dr. Szatkowski serves on national committees for the American Academy of Orthopaedic Surgeons (AAOS), the Orthopaedic Trauma Association (OTA), and the American Orthopaedic Foot and Ankle Society (AOFAS). His active participation in these organizations demonstrates his commitment to shaping the future of orthopaedic surgery. Moreover, as a founding member of Orthobullets, an online orthopaedic educational community, Dr. Szatkowski plays a pivotal role in the education and professional development of orthopaedic surgeons worldwide. This involvement underscores his dedication to patient care and the continuous learning and advancement of the orthopaedic community.

Contents

Preface

Fracture care is an ever-evolving discipline of medicine with rapidly developing new diagnosis methods, treatment recommendations, and innovations in fixation and bone repair. Disability-related fractures throughout all areas of the body affect millions of people worldwide, and the orthopaedic surgeon is tasked with using the latest in evidence-based medicine to improve patient outcomes.

Current Fracture Care is a text that was conceived to gather information on the latest evidence-based practices in fracture care. Chapters have been written by experts from all over the world and have been peer-reviewed prior to publication. I would like to extend a thank you to all the authors who have contributed to this text, as well as the staff at IntechOpen for their support in creating this book.

John T. Riehl
Department of Orthopaedic Surgery,
Medical City UNT/TCU Orthopaedic Surgery Residency Program,
Texas Bone and Joint,
Denton, Texas, USA

Jan P. Szatkowski
Department of Orthopaedic Surgery,
Indiana University Health,
USA

Chapter 1

Recent Advances, Challenges and Future Opportunities for the Use of 3D Bioprinting in Large Bone Defect Treatment

Mostafa Shahrezaee and Ali Zamanian

Abstract

The healing of bone fractures is a well-known physiological process involving various cell types and signaling molecules interacting at the defect site to repair lost bone tissue. However, large bone defects meaning large tissue loss are a complicated problem in orthopedic surgery. In this chapter, we first present the bone treatment procedure and current commonly employed physical and surgical strategies for the treatment of this kind of fracture such as autografts, allografts, xenografts, and synthetic bone grafts as well as tissue engineering techniques. Further to this, we discuss the common limitations that motivate researchers to develop new strategies to overcome these problems. Finally, we will highlight future prospects and novel technologies such as 3D bioprinting which could overcome some of the mentioned challenges in the field of large bone defect reconstruction, with the benefit of fabricating personalized and vascularized medicine.

Keywords: large bone defect (LBd), bone regeneration, tissue engineering, 3D bioprinting, regenerative surgery

1. Introduction

There are 206 bones in human bodies and they consisted of 15% of body weight [1]. Bone defects usually occur by trauma, arthritis, fracture, diseases, etc. and large bone defects need extra intervention to regenerate bone structure and functionality [2]. Bone fractures are very common in societies and around 15.3 million bone fractures with 14 million healthcare visits annually in the United States and it expands with the incensement of the elderly population [3]. The bone defects treatment process can be unsuccessful and lead to delays in treatment, non-unions, and malunions. According to the definition of the Food and Drug Administration (FDA), if the treatment lasts more than 9 months, we are faced with non-unions, but in clinical investigations, this can vary from 2 to 12 months [4]. Considering the high prevalence and the importance of the successfulness of the treatment process, scientists are looking for the best treatment method to treat bone injuries, especially large bone injuries. Today common regeneration replacements are autografts and allografts. Although their limitations such as rare tissue supplements, additional surgeon sites, immunological rejection, and disease transferring restricted their usage. Another treatment method is using implants and bone scaffolds. Although the emergence of tissue engineering in the early 1990s has led to a revolution in bone substitutes, we are facing many challenges in this technique, and efforts must continue to optimize replacement with the highest similarity to natural bone and cartilage tissue [5]. Also, the process of treating bone damage is a complex process that includes various factors. Immune cells and mesenchymal stromal cells (MSCs) cells play an effective role in this process and their behavior should be regulated in such a way that the treatment process is carried out well and does not lead to unwanted reactions such as acute inflammations [6]. Considering the importance of scaffold properties used in cell interactions and as a result in the treatment process, scaffold design should be optimized in such a way that it can provide the desired needs of bone tissue [7]. Recently, 3D printing was introduced as a novel scaffold fabrication method to create a complex cell-laden design with a high mimicking capability of natural tissue using various natural and synthetic materials [8]. Efforts continue to design an ideal scaffold, and perhaps an ideal scaffold for cartilage and bone replacement can be designed in the near future.

In this chapter, the process of bone tissue repair and effective parameters are given first. Then, current used treatment methods and materials for bone tissue repair were summarized. In the following, we will mention the methods of making bone scaffolds based on the 3D printing method and discuss various effective aspects of the 3D printing process, such as the printing methods, the desired needs of the bone scaffolds, and model optimization. Then some of the studies that have been done in this field are discussed. It is hoped that this section can be a guide for researchers in the treatment of bone injuries, especially large bone defects.

2. Regeneration procedure

Replace the entirety of this text with the main body of your chapter. The body is where the author explains experiments, presents and interprets data of one's research. Authors are free to decide how the main body will be structured. However, you are required to have at least one heading. Please ensure that either British or American English is used consistently in your chapter. Since a complete understanding of the bone healing process will help in finding the best bone replacement, this section describes this procedure. Bone healing procedure is a complex process that involves different cellular and molecular events. The bone healing process can be divided into four main steps: (1) hematoma formation, (2) fibrocartilaginous callus formation, (3) bony callus formation, and (4) bone remodeling [9]. This process requires a systematic order and the failure of any of the steps can lead to the failure of the treatment process. The capability of bone regeneration depends on several factors such as the age of the patient, the condition of the patient, the type of bone, the size of the damaged area, the severity of the damage, blood sources, etc. [10]. The bone healing process involves two main pathways: intramembranous (IM) and endochondral (EC) ossification [11].

In the embryo, the endochondral ossification procedure lead to cartilaginous formation as a template and progressive mineralization in long bones [12]. Therefore, as a result, this process is also effective in-directly in bone repair. After the injury during the endochondral ossification process, inflammatory reactions occur between the hematoma at the end of the fracture and its surrounding environment, which results in the creation of temporary granulation tissue, fibrous tissue, and cartilage, and finally, osteoblasts replace the cartilage tissue leads to bone tissue regeneration [13]. Whereas, in intramembranous ossification, the MSCs directly converted to bone cells without cartilage formation [13, 14].

There are various factors such as cell types, growth factors, cytokines, and chemokines that involves in the bone healing process and can facilitate bone healing. Hematoma is the first step of the healing process. It can act as a temporal natural scaffold and some specific cell types such as macrophages and T cells actives at this level and secretes cytokines and begins the regeneration procedure [15]. The acute inflammatory phase usually accelerates in the first 24 hours and finishes 1 week after injury [16]. Chen et al. [17] mentioned Beta-Catenin as an effective signaling in the healing process of bone injuries. This factor acts differently in various levels of fractures. In the first steps, it is necessary for pluripotent mesenchymal cell differentiation to osteoblasts and chondrocytes and after differentiation, it regulates osteoblasts' behaviors.

The secretion of several factors involves in this level includes TNF-Alpha, bone morphogenetic proteins (BMP), tumor necrosis factor-α (TNF-α), interleukin-1 (IL-1), IL-6, IL-11, and IL-18. The secretion of these factors starts angiogenesis [16]. As the healing process continues, chondrocytes, osteoblasts, and endothelial cells are activated and a cartilaginous callus (soft callus) is created to cover the created gap [18]. The regeneration of large bone defects is challenging in surgery and needs extra attention. Infection followed by long bone implant surgery in femoral, tibial, and humeral fractures is another important issue that should be considered. The treatment is performed according to the infection stage. Stage I infections can be treated by antibiotic administration with/without debridement. In Stage II debridement, IM reaming, antibiotic nails, antibiotics can be useful and the stage III infection is usually treated with debridement, exchange nailing, and systemic antibiotic administration [19]. In fact, large bone defects cannot be treated completely without intervention and need extra medical care [20].

3. Bone healing inhibitors

As mentioned above, the process of bone injury regeneration is a complex process that is affected by various factors. In this section, some of the most important negative influencing factors on the bone healing process are mentioned, which should be controlled as much as possible to improve the healing process.

3.1 Non-steroidal anti-inflammatory drugs (NSAID)

Cyclooxygenase (COX) enzymes classified as COX-1 and COX-2, COX-1 is involved in prostaglandins synthesize in physiological conditions. COX-2 is activated in inflammatory conditions and releases prostaglandins. Whereas, NSAIDs inhibit COX activity [21]. The restriction of prostaglandins synthesized with their critical role in osteoblast and osteoclast functions retarded bone regeneration [22]. However, there is a difference of opinion on the use of NSAID and some studies indicate their positive effects on the treatment process. However, it is better to be careful in using this medicine and limit the duration and dosage [23].

3.2 Smoking

It was reported that smoking and its components significantly affect the fracture union especially the tibial shaft fractures, spinal, and foot and ankle fusions. The smokers expressed a 40% increased time to union compared to non-union smokers [24]. Cigarette smoking contains over 4000 toxins such as nicotine, carbon monoxide, nitrosamines, benzenes, aldehydes, and hydrogen cyanide that can inhibit the proliferation of precursor cells, fibroblasts, red blood cells, and macrophages [25].

3.3 Diabetes mellitus

Diabetes mellitus is the other effective factor in bone healing. Diabetes mellitus affects the skeletal system and increases the chance of osteoporosis and fragility fractures, delays bone healing rates, and reduces bone repair quality [26].

4. Different bone defects treatment techniques

There is no standard for the definition of critical-sized bone defects, however typically a defect greater than 1–2 cm or loss over 50% of the circumference of the bone can be called a critical-sized bone defect. It should be notice that this definition also can be changed according to the defect location site or the situation of surrounding soft tissues [27–29]. For example femur, 6–15 cm can be classified as a large bone defect due to its good soft-tissue environment, while tibia defects over 1 cm can be defined as a large bone defect due to its lower healing capacity [27]. In another report, bone defects greater than 3, 5, and 6 cm in the forearm, femur/tibia, and humerus, respectively, were considered critical-sized defects [30]. Therefore, various parameters should be considered in the critical-sized bone defect and in general, it can be defined as an osseous defect that cannot be healed spontaneously during the lifetime or less than 10% of bone regenerated during the lifetime [31]. Different treatment methods have been reported for the treatment of bone complications, especially large bone defects, some of the most important treatment methods are summarized below. **Table 1** summarized the mentioned methods with their advantages and disadvantages.

4.1 Physical treatments

4.1.1 Electrical stimulation

Electrical stimulation can enhance MSCs' adhesion, alignment, division, proliferation, migration, and differentiation [41, 42]. Electrical stimulation can be applied invasive, semi-invasive, or non-invasively. In the invasive method, the DC stimulator electrodes are implanted in the bone injuries and will remove at the end of the regeneration procedure. In the semi-invasive method, the cathodes were placed percutaneously. In the non-invasive method, stimulators were inserted on the skin [43]. Two main mechanisms possibly direct the response of the cells to electrical fields. The first mechanism includes the downstream activation as a consequence of asymmetric redistribution/diffusion of electrically charged surface cell receptors and the other mechanism is attributed to the voltage-gated Ca^{2+} channels activation and the following cellular responses [42].

Treatment method	Categorize	Description	Defect size treatment	Advantages	Disadvantages
Electrical stimulation	Physical treatments	Applying Electrical stimulation to enhance cells differentiation	Low	It can be non-invasive, stimulation of cells proliferation and differentiation	It can be invasive
Low-Intensity pulsed ultrasonography		Applying ultrasound to stimulate cells	Low	Non-invasive	low effectiveness on the pain reduction, poor functional recovery, and poor capability to reduce the recurrent fracture
Extracorporeal shock wave therapy		Applying sequence of high energy acoustic impulses to stimulate cells	Low	Non-invasive, safe, easy, can be applied on most patients	Low efficiency
Ilizarov method	Surgical techniques	applying compression or distraction forces to the bone defects	<9.5 cm [32]	simple, effective, common, minimally invasive	pin tract infection, unconnected bone, re-fracture, bone malformation and transform death
Masquelet -induced membrane		A two-step treatment method with the aim of the soft tissue formation inhibition in the defect site in the first step and bone regeneration in the second step	<25 cm [33]	simple, lower rate of infections	Loosening of the fixation implant, fracture through the graft,and bone resorption.
Autograft	Grafts	a graft of tissue for another site of the same individual's body	<5 cm [34]	High osteoinductive and osteoconductive properties, high success rate, and low probability of immune rejection	Limitation of harvest and formation of secondary surgeon site, fast absorption of autologous
Allograft		non-self-human graft	<3 cm [35]	Providing natural bone structure	risk of disease transmission (HIV, hepatitis B, hepatitis C, and other viruses), and rareness of supplements

Treatment method	Categorize	Description	Defect size treatment	Advantages	Disadvantages
Bone morphogenetic proteins (BMPs)	bioactive molecules, and growth factors	It is a transforming growth factor beta for bone regeneration	<7 cm [36]	high osteogenic potential, FDA approve	side effects such as ectopic osteogenesis, osteolysis, bone cysts, local inflammation, traumatic injuries, postoperative fever, and hemorrhage, or even cancers in excess administration
Statins		3-hydroxy-3-methylglutaryl-coenzyme-A	n.i*	Regulating BMP-2 gene expression and show an osteoinductive role	local retention of the statin
Fibroblast growth factor-2		a famous family member of fibroblast factors	n.i	accelerate cell proliferation, collagen synthesis enhancer, angiogenesis, and osteogenesis	short half-life (3–10 min)
Platelet-Rich Plasma		Using a high concentration of platelets with a lot of therapeutic applications	Cannot be effective in 2.5 cm bone defects [37]	Releasing different growth factors with high regeneration potential	higher infection rate
Insulin-like growth factors		one of the most abundant growth factors in bone matrix	n.i	osteoblasts growth and accelerates bone healing	Not reported
Bisphosphonates		drugs with inhibitory effects on the osteoclasts	n.i	Decrease bone resorption	Increase the risk of fractures and esophageal cancer
dECM		Decellularized natural ECM	n.i	Providing natural ECM structures containing the bone components such as growth factors and cytokines	The possibility of disease transmission
Hydroxyapatite		The main inorganic phase of bones	<10 cm [38] $\leq 15\ cm^3$ [39]	Providing the natural bone component	low dispersibility and tendency to form aggregates

DOI: http://dx.doi.org/10.5772/intechopen.111495

Treatment method	Categorize	Description	Defect size treatment	Advantages	Disadvantages
Cements	Cements	Injectable mixing biomaterial powder with a liquid that can be set in the defect site	<25 cm [40]	Filling complex defects shapes, injectability	thermal necrosis of the bone, cement fragmentation, and foreign body reaction to wear debris
Combination	Combination	Simultaneous usage of different treatment techniques	It depends on the applied techniques	Synergic effects of the used techniques and overcome each other's limitations	It depends on the applied techniques

**No identified range (n.i).*

Table 1.
Comparison of treatment methods for bone injuries along with advantages and disadvantages.

4.1.2 Low-intensity pulsed ultrasonography

Ultrasound treatment is a safe non-invasive method and it was started in the early 1930s for therapy applications [44]. For bone healing Low-Intensity pulsed ultrasonography, the ultrasound is applied every day at 1.5 MHz, with 1 kHz pulse and 30 mW/cm^2 for 20 min time periods [45]. Both bone-forming osteoblasts and mechano-sensitive osteocyte cells can sense the applied ultrasound. Osteoblast accelerates bone formation while regulating inflammatory responses. On the other hand, osteocytes that consisted high percentage of bone cells can sense acoustic radiation force created by ultrasound which leads to biological signals and enhance bone formation [46]. However, some limitation was detected in Low-Intensity pulsed ultrasonography such as low effect on pain reduction, poor functional recovery, and poor capability to reduce recurrent fracture [44].

4.1.3 Extracorporeal shock wave therapy

Extracorporeal shock wave therapy is a non-invasive therapy technique and can be defined as a sequence of high-energy acoustic impulses with a different course that can produce pressure changes while it propagates [47]. This technique has some advantages such as being safe, non-invasive, easy, and can apply to most patients, however, some surgeons believed that it has no significant difference from a placebo [48]. While it was demonstrated that extracorporeal shock wave therapy can be involved in the activation of various biochemical signals that trigger neoangiogenesis, fibroblast proliferation, collagen synthesis, and finally tissue regeneration. On the other hand, the negative phase of the shocks can enhance cell membrane permeability and inhibit calcification deposits and reduce pain [49]. The involved cellular signaling pathways during extracorporeal shock wave therapy are focal adhesion kinase, Extracellular-signal-regulated kinase, Wnt/β-catenin, Protein kinase R-like endoplasmic reticulum kinase/activated transcription factor, ATP/P2X7, Brain-derived neurotrophic factor [50].

4.2 Surgical techniques

Ilizarov method is a simple, effective, common, minimally invasive external fixation technique based on applying compression or distraction forces to the bone defects due to osteogenesis induced by tension stress [51]. Although the Ilizarov method is an applicable technique, especially for large bone defects, in some cases it may be associated with dissatisfaction such as pin tract infection, unconnected bone, re-fracture, bone malformation and transform death reported [52, 53]. One of the other popular surgical methods especially in large bone defects is Masquelet induced membrane [54]. This procedure includes two main steps: first, the created cavity is carefully debridement then is filled with polymethyl methacrylate cement to produce a membrane and inhibit soft tissue formation. In the second step, the cement is removed and the iliac crest cancellous bone or RIA (Reamer-Irrigator-Aspirator) cancellous bone is used to fill the cavity [54, 55].

4.3 Using grafts, bioactive molecules, growth factors, and cement for bone regeneration

4.3.1 Autograft

The gold standard and first bone replacements is autologous bone due to its high osteoinductive and osteoconductive properties [56]. The autografts contain natural bone contents such as bone cells, growth factors, and natural extracellular matrix components such as collagen, non-collagenous proteins, and hydroxyapatite [56]. Although this method has good benefits, it also comes with challenges, for example, a secondary operation that causes suffering for the patient or limitations in the dimensions of the harvested bone, and fast absorption of autologous implant that should be regulated [57].

4.3.2 Allograft

Allografts are non-self-human that can be used as the other option for use in bone defects treatment and consist of one-third of all-bone grafts in North America [58]. The osteoinductivity and mechanical properties of the allograft can be reduced during the freezing, and sterilization processes, while the ECM can provide a natural scaffold for bone regeneration [59]. The main restriction of allografts is the risk of disease transmission (HIV, hepatitis B, hepatitis C, and other viruses), and the rareness of supplements [60].

4.3.3 Bone morphogenetic proteins (BMPs)

BMPs are the most popular subfamily of transforming growth factor beta that are necessary for fetal tissue development and fracture healing [61]. Bone morphogenetic protein-2 (BMP-2) shows high osteogenic potential and can be applied in bone regeneration [62]. It is the only osteoinductive growth factor with FDA approval for clinical usage, but its administration should be controlled. Excess administrated BMPs, especially in the first levels of bone mineralization can cause different side effects such as ectopic osteogenesis, osteolysis, bone cysts, local inflammation, traumatic injuries, postoperative fever, hemorrhage, or even cancers [63].

4.3.4 Statins

Statins, 3-hydroxy-3-methylglutaryl-coenzyme-A, are a family class of drugs reductase inhibitors, with impressive impact on the bone healing procedure. This can be due to the BMP-2 bone factor induction that can facilitate bone healing [64]. The most famous member of this group for bone regeneration applications is Simvastatin [65]. Simvastatin can accelerate bone regeneration by regulating BMP-2 gene expression and show an osteoinductive role through the Ras signaling pathway, and activate mitogen-activated protein kinases. Also, it can inhibit bone density reduction using estrogen receptor-alpha or BMP-2 induction [66, 67]. Feng et al. [68] demonstrated the capability of simvastatin to enhance osteoblast differentiation of mesenchymal stem cells in osteoporosis Sprague–Dawley rats. In another study, Shahrezaee et al. [69] investigated and compared the systemic delivery of atorvastatin, simvastatin, and lovastatin on bone healing. For this purpose, the drugs were orally administrated to the thirty ovariectomized female Sprague–Dawley rats, and the results were analyzed after 60 days. According to the achievements, atorvastatin had no significant effect on bone density, while simvastatin and lovastatin enhanced calcium levels, osteogenic gene expression, bone density, and biomechanical properties. The CT scan of different analyzed groups is shown in **Figure 1 (A-E)** and can prove the better function of simvastatin and lovastatin. In comparison, the simvastatin-treated sample showed a significantly higher resemblance to normal groups and demonstrated increased osteogenic genes and better biomechanical performance.

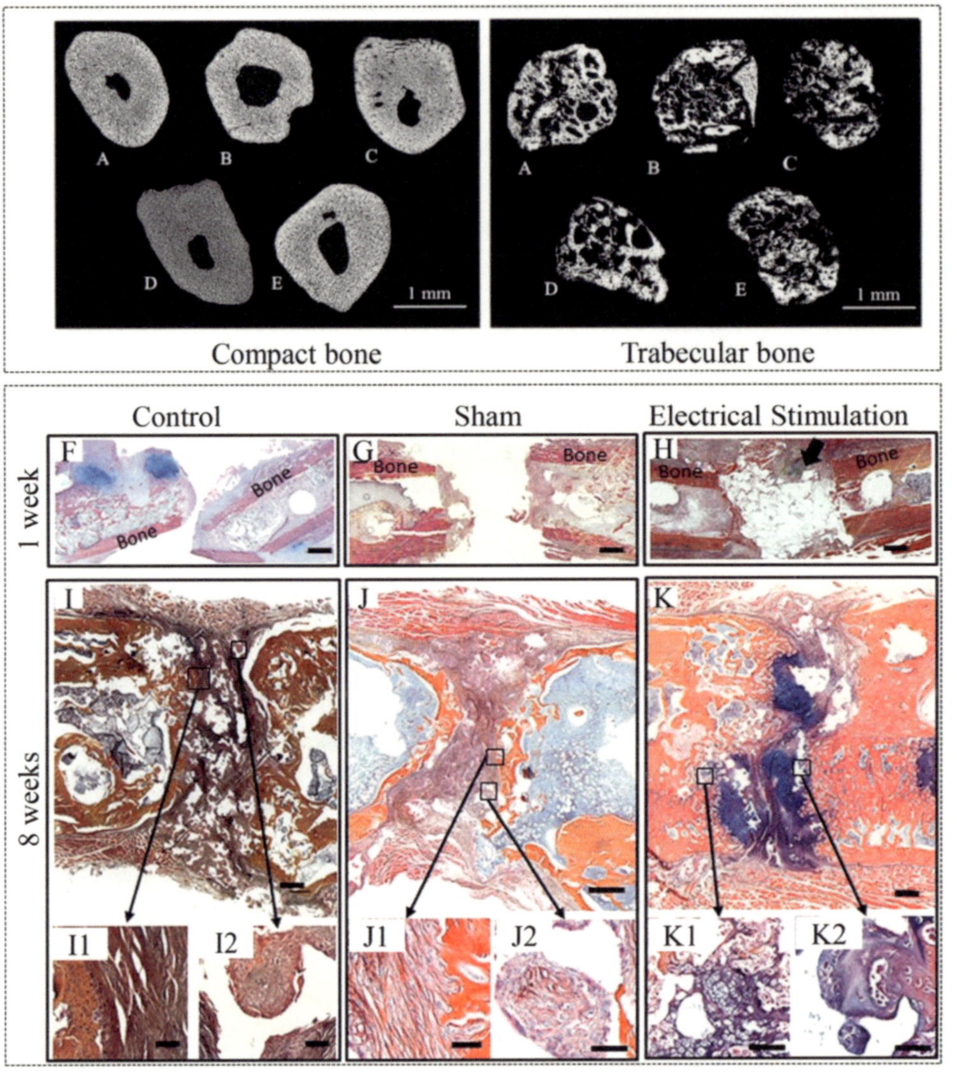

Figure 1.
(A-E): Micro CT results of different analyzed groups after 60 days: (a): Normal, (B): Negative control, (C): Simvastatin, (D): Lovastatin, (E): Atorvastatin [69]. (F-K): The histological investigation of three control (F), sham (G), and experimental (H) groups after 1 week and control (I), sham (J), and experimental (K) groups after 8 weeks. The bottom images are the higher magnifications: (I1) fibrous connective tissue of control, (I2) control scaffolds covered with fibrous, (J1) fibrous connective tissue of sham, (J2) sham scaffolds covered with mixed tissue, (K1) cartilage and bone tissue of experimental group, (K2) experimental group covered with cartilage and bone tissue [70].

4.3.5 Fibroblast growth factor-2

Fibroblast growth factor-2 is a famous family member of fibroblast factors with unique properties such as mitotic promoters that can accelerate cell proliferation, collagen synthesis enhancer, angiogenesis, and osteogenesis [71]. However, its short half-life (3–10 min) should be regulated using different drug release carriers because excess Fibroblast growth factor-2 usage can cause side effects and depressant bone regeneration [72].

4.3.6 Platelet-rich plasma

Platelet-Rich Plasma (PRP) refers to the high concentration of platelets (two to five higher than blood) in a small volume of plasma with a lot of therapeutic applications due to the capability of platelets to secret different growth factors [73]. It was reported that approximately 300 bioactive cytokines exist in PRP and their release can trigger various cellular interactions and facilitate tissue regeneration. Although there is no international protocol for PRP usage [74]. The main growth factors are platelet-derived growth factor (PDGFaa, PDGFbb, PDGFab), TGFβ1/TGFβ2, VEGF, FGF, epithelial growth factor (EGF), bone morphogenetic protein (BMP), hepatocyte growth factor (HGF) and insulin-like growth factor (IGF) [75]. These growth factors can modulate inflammation, accelerate cell proliferation and differentiation, promote angiogenesis, and as a result accelerate bone regeneration [76]. The performance of PRP in large bone treatment is successful with a lower rate of pain score and shorter healing duration. However, a higher infection rate was reported [77].

4.3.7 Insulin-like growth factors

Insulin-like growth factor-1 (IGF-1) is one of the most abundant growth factors in bone matrix with a wide range of physiological functions [78]. The administration of IGF-1 lead to enhance osteoblasts growth and accelerate bone healing [79]. IGF receptor is a cell surface receptor named an Insulin-like growth factor 1 receptor and after binding to Insulin-like growth factors, it activates two main signaling pathways: the phosphoinositide 3-kinase (PI3 K)/AKT and the RAS/mitogen-activated protein kinase (MAPK) and leads to promoting cell proliferation, migration, and proliferation [80]. In addition to IGF-1, metformin can improve osteogenic differentiation and facilitate bone regeneration [81]. Shahrezaei et al. [82] reported that metformin coating of poly (lactic acid) and polycaprolactone scaffold increased the osteogenic and angiogenic markers expressions and accelerated the regeneration of rats' large bone defects.

4.3.8 Bisphosphonates

Bisphosphonates are drugs with inhibitory effects on the osteoclasts using increasing their apoptosis rate of them and interfering with resorption signals sent from the bone matrix [83]. These drugs are classified into two main categories with different mechanisms: nitrogen-containing bisphosphonates, and non-nitrogen-containing bisphosphonates. The non-nitrogen ones metabolized to analogs of adenosine triphosphate and interfere with mitochondrial activity and lead to cell death, while the nitrogen-containing ones inhibit farnesyl pyrophosphate synthase which can be effective in protein transportation and lead to cell death and inhibit osteoclast maturation [84].

4.3.9 dECM

The extracellular matrix (ECM) is a complex structure with various components including collagen, glycosaminoglycans, chondroitin sulfate, elastin, etc. [85]. In the decellularization procedure of ECM, the cells were eliminated with low harm to the natural structure and components of the ECM [85, 86]. Decellularized extracellular matrix (dECM) derived from natural ECM can be used as a biomaterial in tissue engineering applications [87]. The dECM introduces a natural structure for bone replacement containing the bone components such as growth factors and cytokines [88]. Also, dECM can provide cellular activities that are necessary for bone healing [89].

4.3.10 Hydroxyapatite

Natural bone ECM consists of organic and inorganic phases and the base of the organic phase is calcium phosphate, especially hydroxyapatite [90]. Therefore, hydroxyapatite is one of the most studied materials in bone regeneration applications [91–94]. The hydroxyapatite can be used alone, synthetically, porously, in a resorbable form, or combined with natural or synthetic materials such as β-TCP, PRP, collagen, and bioactive glass [95]. Walsh et al. [96] showed a high potential of hydroxyapatite-collagen scaffold for the treatment of critical-sized bone defects with 28-fold and 7-fold increments in the bone volume and new bone area after 4 weeks.

4.3.11 Cements

Cement is used clinically due to its injection capability and molding as a paste and filling the irregular bone defects in a minimally invasive manner [97]. The Cement is obtained by mixing biomaterial powder with a liquid that can be set when injected into the defect site [98]. Polymethyl methacrylate is one of the common cement to repair bone defects [99]. Jia et al. [100] demonstrated the positive application of antibiotic PMMA cement (0.5 g of gentamicin per 40 g of PMMA) coating on the locking plates for infection inhabitation and enhancing bone regeneration. On the other hand, self-setting calcium phosphate is the other common type of cement with a lot of applications. These cements provide injectibility with favorable bone defect-filling capability [101].

4.4 Combining techniques

Although each of the treatment methods mentioned above has benefits and potential effects, however, all methods face limitations. The simultaneous use and combination of the mentioned methods to provide a new treatment method can lead to the simultaneous use of the benefits of each method in such a way that they overcome each other's limitations. Leppik et al. [70] proposed a combined technique for the treatment of large bone defects by using tissue engineering and electrical stimulation. For this purpose, the test was analyzed *in-vitro* and *in-vivo*. The *in-vivo* experiment was performed on three different groups: large femur-defected rats treated with β -TCP scaffolds (control group), β-TCP scaffolds and Adipose tissue-derived mesenchymal stem cells (AT-MSC) (sham group), electrical stimulation, β-TCP scaffolds, and Adipose tissue-derived mesenchymal stem cells (experimental group). The 3 cm defects were created in the right limbs of the rats under general anesthesia. After 1 week, Staining was performed using Alcian Blue, Orange-G, and Hematoxylin histological investigation was carried out (**Figure 1 (F-K)**), the 80% defect gap was covered with soft tissue in the experimental group, while there was a high uncovered gap was seen in the control and sham groups. Although there can be a better condition in the sham group in comparison with control samples. After 8 weeks, histological observations showed that cartilage and bone tissue were formed properly in the experimental group.

In another combined treatment method, Qi et al. [78] used Electrical stimulation and insulin-like growth factor-1 (IGF-1) for bone regeneration. The effect of this method was tested on MC3T3-E1 cell behavior and the results were analyzed with different techniques. According to the achievements, the combination of electrical stimulation and IGF-1 acted synergistically and lead to higher expression of osteogenic marker genes and alkaline phosphatase activity, and cell mineralization. The results of alizarin red staining of the cell mineralization were shown in **Figure 2 (A-H)**. The combination techniques demonstrated higher calcium content in comparison with the cells that only receive the IGF-1 factor. On the other hand, when the concentration of IGF-1 was 100 and 200 ng/ml a higher calcium content was detected. In another clinical trial, Combal et al. [102] combined the Masquelet-Induced Membrane and Capanna Vascularized Fibula with an Allograft large femoral bone defects and introduced it as Capasquelet. The technique can be used for the treatment of bone defects with at least 10 cm loss. For this purpose, four patients suffering from tumors/traumatic bone defects were operated on with this combination technique. The result proved the important effect of the induced membrane in the regeneration process with fast allograft and fibula union and early weight-bearing **Figure 2 (I-J)**.

4.5 Novel techniques

4.5.1 Cell therapy

Few cell types can form heterotrophic bones while many cell types can create mineralized tissues [103]. Progenitor cells are the best cell population for cell therapy applications. The number of the needed cells depends on different factors such as bone fracture types and size, cell source, therapeutic method, and biomaterials, whereas usually for a 4 cm large bone defect approximately 600 million cells are sufficient [104]. Mesenchymal stem cells are extensively studied in bone regeneration with favorable clinical application, especially in dental and orthopedic fields [105]. Furthermore, MSCs can regulate physical contact between cells and enhance cell–cell interactions for osteogenesis [106]. Although these cells can be isolated from different parts of the body, the gold standard is included bone marrow-derived MSCs (BM-MSCs) due to their easiness and high osteogenic capacity [107]. BMSCs are the most popular cell population for bone treatment over 50 years ago [104]. In the Hernigou process, the bone marrow aspirates to the bone defect sites [106]. Furthermore, the infusion of BMSCs is used for the treatment of children with severe osteogenesis imperfect [108].

4.5.2 Tissue engineering

The limitations of the previous bone replacements such as donor-site scarcity, high risk of disease transmission, and immune rejection made the scientists find a new solution. Tissue engineering introduced promising strategies for bone regeneration [109–111].

Tissue engineering consisted of cells, scaffolds, and bioactive molecules. Both natural and synthetic materials can be used for scaffold fabrication in tissue engineering with their unique properties. Natural materials provide better biological recognition and cellular interactions [112]. Synthetic materials can be modified according to the requirements and the source is usually abundant. On the other hand, the material

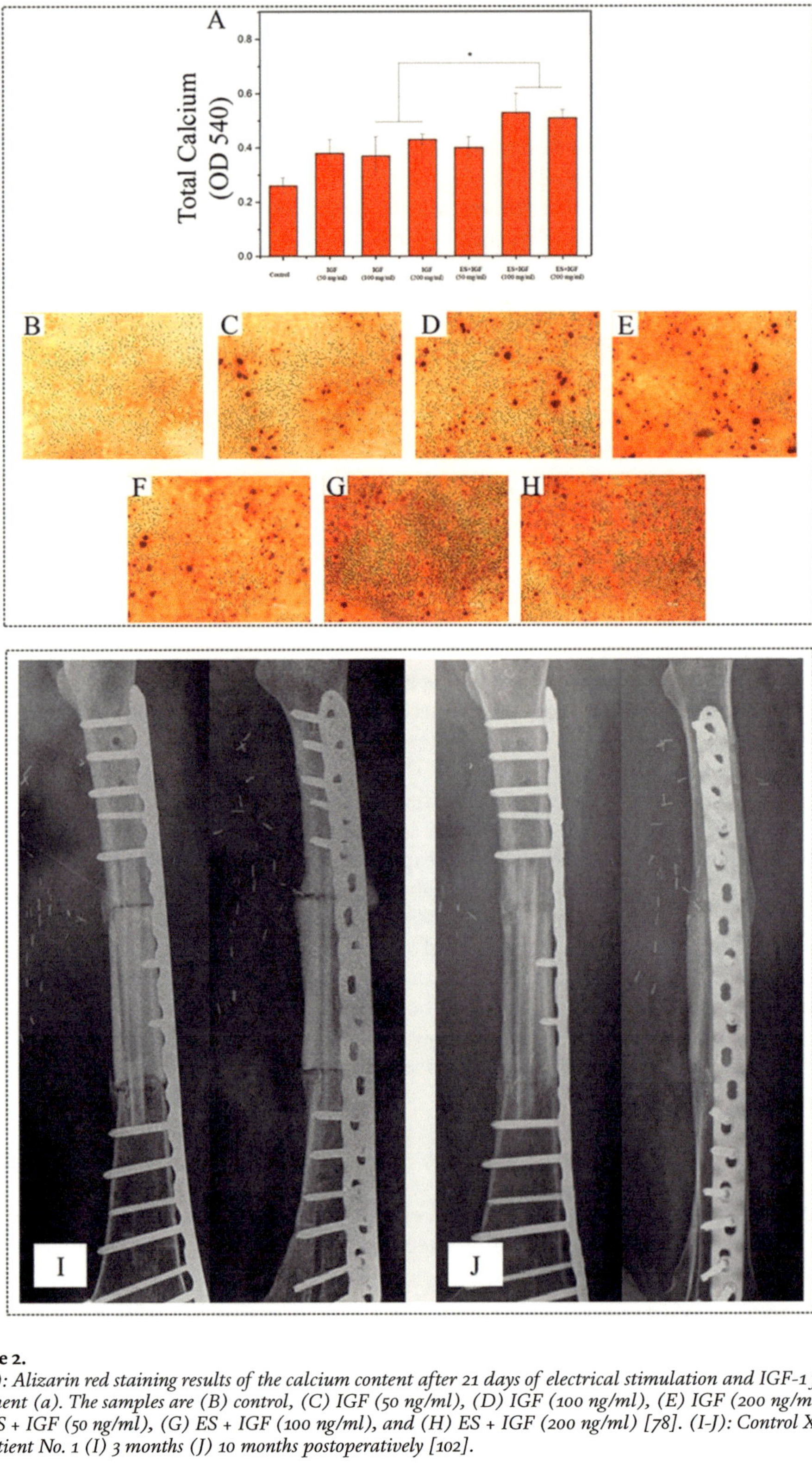

Figure 2.
(A-H): Alizarin red staining results of the calcium content after 21 days of electrical stimulation and IGF-1 factor treatment (a). The samples are (B) control, (C) IGF (50 ng/ml), (D) IGF (100 ng/ml), (E) IGF (200 ng/ml), (F) ES + IGF (50 ng/ml), (G) ES + IGF (100 ng/ml), and (H) ES + IGF (200 ng/ml) [78]. (I-J): Control X-rays for patient No. 1 (I) 3 months (J) 10 months postoperatively [102].

should be modified to overcome usual synthetic materials disadvantages such as low material-tissue integrity, low vascularization, poor cell attachment, and therefore functional bone regeneration [113, 114].

5. Specific bone scaffolds requirements

The scaffold is one of the key elements of tissue engineering that provide mechanical support for cell adhesion and growth [115]. To design an ideal scaffold material selection, scaffold architecture, and scaffold fabrication techniques create important roles [116]. Bone scaffolds should provide a high porosity for cell adhesion, proliferation, and growth; meanwhile providing adequate mechanical properties during bone regeneration [117, 118]. It was suggested 75–95 vol% porosity is proper for bone scaffolds [119]. The osteoblast cells are in the range of 10–50 μm and prefer the larger pore size (100–200 μm) for growth and mineralization that could allow the penetration of macrophages, cell migration, and vascularization. Whereas lower pore size of this range leads to the creation of fibrous tissue and inhibits bone tissue regeneration [120].

The other important parameter for designing scaffolds is the swelling ratio. There are various properties affecting the swelling ratio such as hydrophilicity, cross-link density, porosity, pH, and the environmental characteristics [121–124]. A high swelling ratio facilitates fluid penetration and as a result enhances nutrition, oxygen, and waste material transportation, while the structures with an excess swelling ratio usually do not show adequate mechanical properties for bone healing [125]. The range of mechanical properties depends on the bone type, however, in general for elastic modulus range is reported 18.6 ± 28.8 GPa and 10–157 MPa for cortical and cancellous bone, respectively [126]. Therefore, it is expected the designed scaffold could provide sufficient mechanical properties for bone tissue during the regeneration procedure. Furthermore, the biodegradation ratio of the construct scaffolds should match the tissue growth rate [127]. Each bone requires a specific degradation ratio for example in spinal fusion regeneration it needs 9 months while it is suggested 3–6 months for craniomaxillofacial healing [119].

6. Scaffolds fabrication methods

Scaffolds act as a temporal template for cell attachments and growth that can contain different cell types, growth factors, drugs, and bioactive molecules. Although the material selection had a great impact on the scaffolds' properties, the scaffold's fabrication technique is also an important criterion. There are different techniques for scaffold fabrication such as gas-foaming, phase separation, particle leaching, electrospinning, freeze-drying, freeze-casting, and 3D bio-printing. An ideal scaffold should be able to create the most similar structure to the natural bone tissue along the same physical, chemical, and biological properties while providing reproducibility with minimal cost and time. The conventional scaffold fabrication methods showed poor controllability during the creation process to fabricate complex structures with tunable micro-scale and macro-scale. The recent scaffold fabrication methods such as 3D bio-printing allow high controllability, the capability of complex structures, and the inclusion of the cells and growth factors in the structure [128–130].

6.1 Three dimensional bio-printing

Recently, 3D bio-printing is introduced as a novel scaffold fabrication method and has provided numerous capabilities compared to the traditional methods such as a lower rate of residual organic solvents which decreases the harmful effects of these chemical solvents on the cell's survival and interactions, or scaffold designing before printing which leads to personalization [131, 132]. Also, it is possible to build complex structures with/without cells [133]. The most important benefit of 3D bio-printing for bone tissue engineering is controlling cell distribution [134]. The printing materials that contain cells are called 'bio-ink' and should demonstrate some features for cell survival and the creation of a favorable bone substitute. The most important features in the bio-inks selection are biocompatibility, printability, fidelity, viscoelasticity, shear-thinning, yield stress, shelf life, cross-linking capability, and even cost [135].

6.1.1 Methods

In the first years of the emergence of 3D printing, conventional methods of this technique such as fused deposition modeling (FDM), stereolithography (SLA), and selective laser sintering (SLS) were used to print tissue engineering structures. Although these methods provided unique capabilities compared to the traditional scaffold construction methods, however, as time passed and the disadvantages of these methods became clear, such as the inability to load cells and bioactive molecules, the inadequate resolution, and the impossibility of using a wide range of materials led researchers to develop 3D bio-printing technology. In recent years, the use of 3D bio-printing technology has accelerated. This method is divided into three main types: inkjet-based bioprinting, extrusion-based bioprinting, and laser-assisted bioprinting [136–139]. Inkjet-based bioprinting includes the deposition of bio-ink droplets onto a substrate. Although this method can print a cell-laden scaffold at a high speed, the number of biomaterials that can be used in an inkjet printer is limited, due to the rapid gelation time requirement. The extrusion-based bioprinting method is extruding high cell density laden bio-inks to create scaffold structures. It is the most easiest and popular 3D bio-printing method. In laser-assisted bioprinting, the bio-inks are printed using the laser in a nozzle-free manner with higher resolution. The laser heats the determined points and deposits the cells in the exact place [140].

6.1.2 Bone model optimizing

As mentioned before, the 3D bio-printing can create personalized complex structures. The computer modeling of the 3D bio-printing structures has two main steps. The first step is data acquisition using computed tomography (CT) or magnetic resonance imaging (MRI) and the second step is image processing and model generation [141]. The 3D models should be predictable and shows controllable shape change. Therefore, the 3D model design should be optimized by considering chemical composition, volume fraction, and structural features such as pore size, pore shape, pore distributions, and mechanical properties [142]. The finite element analysis can be used to calculate the mechanical properties of the designed structures and predict the results, theoretically. Liang et al. [143] demonstrated the tetragonal structures showed better mechanics than the tetragonal, hexagonal, and wheel-like designed structures for bone replacements using finite element analysis and an electromechanical universal testing system. The combination of state-of-the-art optimization techniques with computer models can provide a basis for predicting scaffold behavior and optimizing the designed scaffolds for bone regeneration, especially for large bone defect regeneration [144].

7. The previous studies on large bone treatment using 3D bio-printing

Pitaco et al. [145] developed a hypertrophic cartilage graft for the replacement of critical-sized defects. The bio-ink was prepared with Human mesenchymal stem/stromal cells loading in the fibrin-based bio-ink and 3D bio-printing was performed in the polycaprolactone framework. The designed constructs were implanted into nude mice and expressed a high potential for bone remodeling with high efficiency in vascularization and bone formation. In another trial Sun et al. [146] introduced a multi-component bio-ink for the treatment of critical-sized bone defects in diabetes mellitus patients. The gelatin, gelatin methacryloyl, and 4-arm poly (ethylene glycol) acrylate bio-ink were loaded with BMSCs, RAW264.7 macrophages, and BMP-4-loaded mesoporous silica nanoparticles. Silica nanoparticles could enhance the mechanical stability and control the release of BMP-4. The existence of BMP-4 led to the polarization of RAW264.7 to M2 macrophages to produce BMP-2 and anti-inflammatory factors and the dual presence of BMP-2 and BMP-4 facilitated the osteogenic differentiation of BMSCs. Zhang et al. [147] developed a human mesenchymal stem cell-laden graphene oxide/alginate/gelatin bio-ink with different concentrations of graphene oxide (0.5, 1, and 2 mg/ml) to create bone scaffolds. The results demonstrated that the scaffolds containing 1 mg/ml graphene oxide had higher shape fidelity, osteogenic differentiation, and mineral volume for mimicking critical-sized calvarial bone defects. Furthermore, Dong et al. [148] evaluated the rabbit bone marrow mesenchymal stem cells and bone morphogenetic protein-2 encapsulated chitosan hydrogel in 3D printed polycaprolactone scaffolds with the aim of bone tissue regeneration. The cellular investigation after 2 weeks confirmed high osteogenesis and bone matrix formation of the proposed scaffold. Khoshnood et al. [149] introduced a novel 3D bio-printed composition for bone regeneration. According to their study, printing 1 wt % tragacanth and 3 wt % alginate bio-ink can provide favorable printability and viscosity. The addition of tragacanth to the alginate modulates the biodegradation ratio to 21 days. Furthermore, adding hydroxyapatite improved osteoconductivity. The prepared bio-inks provided high cell differentiation support with the expression of CD105, CD44, and CD90 surface markers. Hao et al. [150] clinically investigated the printing capacity to treat complicated and large acetabular bone defects. The personalized titanium prosthesis was designed based on computed tomography and X-ray and the final model was achieved using Siemens NX software and Magics software and then the printing was performed. After this step, the prosthesis was trimmed, polished, sandblasted, and cleaned. Then, a surgical process was performed. According to the radiographic and software analysis, the 3D-printed prosthesis showed a high Harris hip score recovery rate in all patients. Wang et al. [151] used 3D-printed polylactic acid (PLA) and nano-hydroxyapatite scaffolds for large bone treatment. The polymeric part was used to provide the required mechanical and degradation rate of the bone scaffolds and nano-hydroxyapatite was added to provide osteoconductivity and improve the load-bearing capacity. The prepared scaffolds were tested *in-vivo* in the rabbit model. The high biocompatibility and osteogenic properties proved the high potential of these scaffolds for further future studies. Li et al. [152] introduced bio-active 3D printed scaffolds for the regeneration of large and load-bearing bone defects. The scaffolds compound was strontium-hardystonite-gahnite and the scaffolds were tested in the large bone-sized defects of the sheep tibia for 3 and 12 months. Mathematical modeling confirmed and highlighted the importance of the surgical process and implant fixation as much as the implant compositions and the *in-vivo* results revealed high induction of bone formation after 12 months.

7.1 *In-situ* printing

In-situ printing or *in-vivo* 3D bio-printing is defined as the direct printing of bio-inks at the defects' site with the aim of creating or repairing damaged tissue in a clinical setting. In this procedure, the robotic arms are assembled with the bio-printing unit, and the printing is conducted in minimally invasive routes in the defect site [153]. Cohen et al. [154] used in-situ bio-printing for the treatment of osteochondral defects. The alginate and demineralized bone matrix were printed using a built-in-house extrusion-based bio-printer for this purpose. Two types of defects were created in the calf femur: a cartilage only and an osteochondral defect. The results demonstrated the high geometric precision of the in-situ printing process. In another study, Kerique et al. [155] in situ printed the Nano-hydroxyapatite in the mouse calvaria defect model using a laser printer. They suggested that the in-situ printing usage by surgeons or actual robots can reduce the used materials to pL volume and the spatial resolution increased. In another trial on the robotic *in-situ* bio-printing for large bone healing, Li et al. [156] presented a new method for optimizing robotic printing. The extrusion-based bio-printer was selected due to the easier structural and mechanical controllability and a modified 4-DOF robot with higher kinematic accuracy of 0.5 mm was used. The bio-printing was performed using a double-network hydrogel bio-ink consisting of alginate, polyethene glycol diacrylate (PEGDA), and methacrylated gelatin (GelMA). Alginate was cross-linked with calcium ions and PEGDA and GelMA created a covalently cross-linked network. The in-vivo successful results on the large tibia bone defects of pigs revealed the high potential of this method for future clinical applications of *in-situ* large bone regeneration.

7.2 Pre-vascular scaffolds

Angiogenesis is an important factor in the bone healing process in both intramembranous and endochondral ossification healing ways [157]. In endochondral ossification cartilaginous continues in the vascular network and the network provides cell sources, nutrition, oxygen, and growth factors needed for the repair process, and then osseous tissue formed [18]. Osteogenesis is closely related to angiogenesis during neo-bone tissue formation [158]. Therefore, efforts to create pre-vascular structures in order to create fully functional and perfusable tissue constructs for clinical applications have been made with the help of 3D bio-printing [159]. Kuss et al. [160] designed a pre-vascularized scaffold with the co-culture of Human adipose-derived mesenchymal stem cells (ADMSC) and human umbilical vein endothelial cells (HUVEC) on the polycaprolactone/hydroxyapatite scaffolds. Then, the pre-vascularized scaffolds were implanted in the nude mice, and vascularization capacity was analyzed. The results confirmed the microvessel and lumen formation and increased the vascular network formation. In addition, Nulty et al. [161] implanted the prevascularized 3D-printed polycaprolactone scaffolds to treat critical-size bone defects. The prevascularization was performed using both human bone marrow stem/stromal cells (hBMSCs) and human umbilical vein endothelial cells (HUVEC) in a fibrin base bio-ink. The *in-vivo* results showed increased vascularization and as a result bone regeneration.

7.3 Osteochondral scaffolds

Osteoarthritis is the most prevalent joint disease that affects millions of people around the world. The growing elderly population increases its prevalence and needs extra attention [162]. The avascular nature and rare source of repair cells lead to the restricted self-regeneration capability of cartilage [163] and existing treatment methods mostly repair single cartilage tissue and are not suitable for the whole osteochondral replacement [164]. As a result, the search for the best osteochondral substitute continues.

A study by Gardner et al. [165] investigated the composition and the porosity of the clinically available polycaprolactone (PCL) and β -tricalcium phosphate (β-TCP) and proposed the selected scaffold for intervertebral disc replacement. The results demonstrated that β-TCP facilitated the proliferation and differentiation of the C3H10 cells. According to the results, the design consisted of 45% porous material with 60% of β-TCP for the topper and lower parts and the core consisted of polycaprolactone with 70–75% porosity to stimulate the cartilage section of the intervertebral disc (**Figure 3 (A-B)**). In another study, Kilian et al. [166] introduced a novel combination

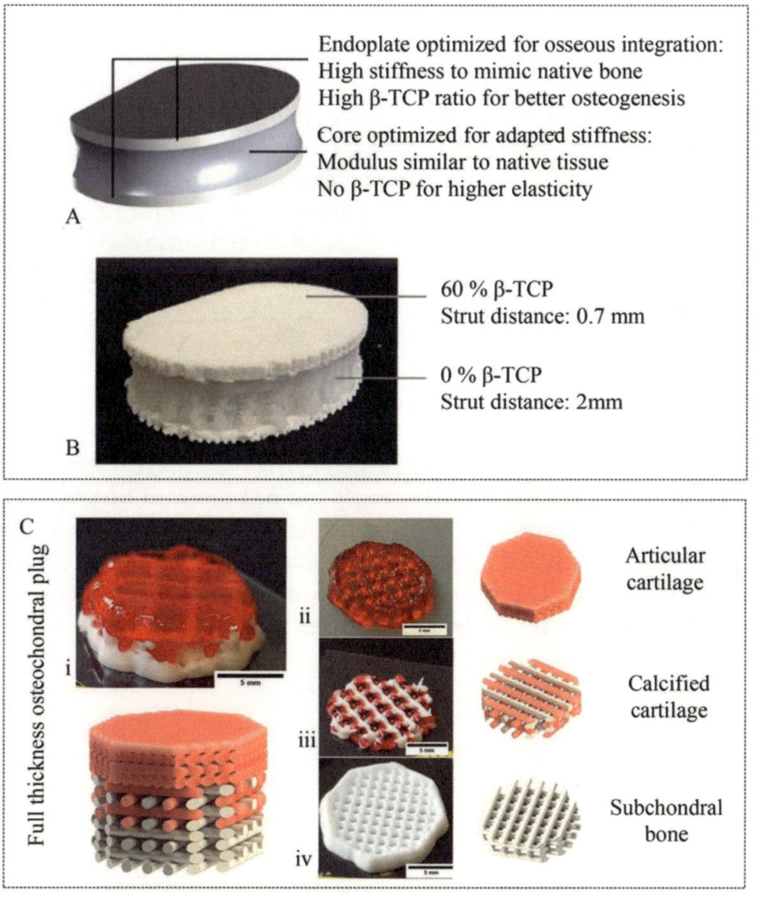

Figure 3.
(A-B): Novel 3D printed polycaprolactone and b-tricalcium phosphate (β-TCP) scaffold for intervertebral disc replacement [165]. (C) the multi-component 3D plotted scaffolds designed by Kilian et al. [166] for osteochondral treatment consisted of three main parts to stimulate natural osteochondral structures.

for osteochondral bio-printing. The bio-ink included the alginate-methylcellulose with calcium phosphate cement. The multi-channel 3D plotted structure consisted of three parts. The upper part contained the hMSC cell-laden hydrogel and partly mineralized calcium phosphate cement. The middle part was a biphasic interwoven network of both hMSC cell-laden hydrogel and calcium phosphate cement to mimic calcified cartilage and the bottom part was the subchondral bone that was created using pure calcium phosphate cement (**Figure 3 (C)**). The results demonstrated high efficiency of cell survival with the potential of redifferentiation to produce cartilage extracellular matrix (ECM) components.

Shim et al. [167] described a 3D bio-printed construct with different ECM types for osteochondral tissue engineering. The bio-ink was constructed on the base of atelocollagen and supramolecular hyaluronic acid loaded with human mesenchymal stromal cells. The mixture of Cucurbit[6]uril/conjugated HA and 1,6-diaminohexane -conjugated HA ledto creating a biphasic stable construct without the need for chemical cross-linker and physical stimuli. The designed scaffolds were tested in the knee joint of rabbits and showed remarkable osteochondral regeneration after 8 weeks.

8. Future direction and conclusion

Bone regeneration is a very complex process that includes various factors, cells, and biomolecules. In large bone defects, the body does not have the ability to heal these injuries by itself. As a result, it needs external interventions. Although extensive methods, including surgical methods and physical methods using different materials, are used to treat bone injuries today, these methods face limitations. The spread of bone diseases with the increase in the elderly population leads researchers to create alternative treatment methods for bone healing. Recently, 3D bio-printing has been proposed for the treatment of large bone injuries, and extensive research has been done in this field in the last few years. This study shows the potential of 3D bio-printing strategies in the creation of different scaffolds for large bone tissue defect regeneration. The use of printed scaffolds containing cells with the ability to imitate natural tissue has opened a window of hope for creating new bone substitutes. Innovation in the use of these methods, such as in-situ printing, pre-vascularization, or the use of multi-matrix scaffolds for the combined treatment of bone and cartilage increases the capability of these structures. There is still a need to investigate and create new scaffolds in this field, which can increase the therapeutic potential of these scaffolds in the future. It seems that 3D bio-printing can provide effective treatment methods for repairing large bone tissues in the near future.

Author details

Mostafa Shahrezaee[1]* and Ali Zamanian[2]

1 Faculty of Medicine, Department of Orthopedic Surgery, AJA University of Medical Science, Tehran, Iran

2 Biomaterials Research Group, Nanotechnology and Advanced Materials Department, Materials and Energy Research Center (MERC), Tehran, Iran

*Address all correspondence to: moshahrezayee@yahoo.com

References

[1] Aidun A, Zamanian A, Ghorbani F. Immobilization of polyvinyl alcohol-siloxane on the oxygen plasma-modified polyurethane-carbon nanotube composite matrix. Journal of Applied Polymer Science. 2020;**137**(12):1-12

[2] Ghorbani F, Zamanian A, Behnamghader A, Daliri JM. A novel pathway for in situ synthesis of modified gelatin microspheres by silane coupling agents as a bioactive platform. Journal of Applied Polymer Science. 2018;**135**(41):1-10

[3] Pivonka P, Dunstan CR. Role of mathematical modeling in bone fracture healing. Bonekey Reports. 2012;**1**(October):1-10. DOI: 10.1038/bonekey.2012.221

[4] Buza J. Bone healing in 2016. Clinical Cases in Mineral and Bone Metabolism. 2016;**13**(2):101-105

[5] Liu M, Zeng X, Ma C, Yi H, Ali Z, Mou X, et al. Injectable hydrogels for cartilage and bone tissue engineering. Bone Research. 2017;**5**:17014

[6] Maruyama M, Rhee C, Utsunomiya T, Zhang N, Ueno M, Yao Z, et al. Modulation of the inflammatory response and bone healing. Frontiers in Endocrinology (Lausanne). 2020;**11**:386

[7] Zimmerling A, Yazdanpanah Z, Cooper DML, Johnston JD, Chen X. 3D printing PCL/nHA bone scaffolds: Exploring the influence of material synthesis techniques. Biomaterials Research. 2021;**25**(1):3

[8] Wang Z, Wang Y, Yan J, Zhang K, Lin F, Xiang L, et al. Pharmaceutical electrospinning and 3D printing scaffold design for bone regeneration. Advanced Drug Delivery Reviews. 2021;**174**:504-534

[9] Sheen JR, Garla VV. Fracture Healing Overview. Treasure Island (FL): StatPearls; 2021

[10] Fernandez-Yague MA, Abbah SA, McNamara L, Zeugolis DI, Pandit A, Biggs MJ. Biomimetic approaches in bone tissue engineering: Integrating biological and physicomechanical strategies. Advanced Drug Delivery Reviews. 2015;**84**:1-29

[11] Wei S, Ma JX, Xu L, Gu XS, Ma XL. Biodegradable materials for bone defect repair. Military Medical Research. 2020;**7**(1):1-25

[12] Martin I, Wendt D, Heberer M. The role of bioreactors in tissue engineering. Trends in Biotechnology. 2004;**22**(2):80-86

[13] Lopes D, Martins-Cruz C, Oliveira MB, Mano JF. Bone physiology as inspiration for tissue regenerative therapies. Biomaterials. 2018;**185**:240-275

[14] Tortelli F, Tasso R, Loiacono F, Cancedda R. The development of tissue-engineered bone of different origin through endochondral and intramembranous ossification following the implantation of mesenchymal stem cells and osteoblasts in a murine model. Biomaterials. 2010;**31**(2):242-249

[15] Schell H, Duda GN, Peters A, Tsitsilonis S, Johnson KA, Schmidt-Bleek K. The haematoma and its role in bone healing. Journal of Experimental Orthopaedics. 2017;**4**(1):5

[16] Marsell R, Einhorn TA. The biology of fracture healing. Injury. 2011;**42**(6):551-555

[17] Chen Y, Whetstone HC, Lin AC, Nadesan P, Wei Q, Poon R, et al. Beta-catenin signaling plays a disparate role in different phases of fracture repair: Implications for therapy to improve bone healing. PLoS Medicine. 2007;**4**(7):e249

[18] Ghiasi MS, Chen J, Vaziri A, Rodriguez EK, Nazarian A. Bone fracture healing in mechanobiological modeling: A review of principles and methods. Bone Reports. 2017;**6**:87-100

[19] Makridis KG, Tosounidis T, Giannoudis PV. Management of Infection after Intramedullary Nailing of long bone fractures: Treatment protocols and outcomes. The Open Orthopaedics Journal. 2013;**7**(1):219-226

[20] Dennis SC, Berkland CJ, Bonewald LF, Detamore MS. Endochondral ossification for enhancing bone regeneration: Converging native extracellular matrix biomaterials and developmental engineering In vivo. Tissue Engineering. Part B, Reviews. 2015;**21**(3):247-266

[21] Lisowska B, Kosson D, Domaracka K. Positives and negatives of nonsteroidal anti-inflammatory drugs in bone healing: The effects of these drugs on bone repair. Drug Design, Development and Therapy. 2018;**12**:1809-1814

[22] Vuolteenaho K, Moilanen T, Moilanen E. Non-steroidal anti-inflammatory drugs, Cyclooxygenase-2 and the bone healing process. Basic & Clinical Pharmacology & Toxicology. 2007;**102**:10-14

[23] Fader L, Whitaker J, Lopez M, Vivace B, Parra M, Carlson J, et al. Tibia fractures and NSAIDs. Does it make a difference? A multicenter retrospective study. Injury. 2018;**49**(12):2290-2294

[24] Patel RA, Wilson RF, Patel PA, Palmer RM. The effect of smoking on bone healing. Bone and Joint Research. 2013;**2**(6):102-111

[25] Shibli JA, Piattelli A, Iezzi G, Cardoso LA, Onuma T, de Carvalho PSP, et al. Effect of smoking on early bone healing around oxidized surfaces: A prospective, controlled study in human jaws. Journal of Periodontology. 2010;**81**(4):575-583

[26] Hamann C, Picke A-K, Campbell GM, Balyura M, Rauner M, Bernhardt R, et al. Effects of parathyroid hormone on bone mass, bone strength, and bone regeneration in male rats with type 2 diabetes mellitus. Endocrinology. 2014;**155**(4):1197-1206

[27] Schemitsch EH. Size matters: Defining critical in bone defect size! Journal of Orthopaedic Trauma. 2017;**31**(5):S20-S22

[28] Nauth A, Schemitsch E, Norris B, Nollin Z, Watson JT. Critical-size bone defects: Is there a consensus for diagnosis and treatment? Journal of Orthopaedic Trauma. 2018;**32**(3):S7-S11

[29] Mauffrey C, Barlow BT, Smith W. Management of Segmental Bone Defects. The Journal of the American Academy of Orthopaedic Surgeons. 2015;**23**(3):143-153

[30] Calori GM, Mazza E, Colombo M, Ripamonti C. The use of bone-graft substitutes in large bone defects: Any specific needs? Injury. 2011;**42**(Suppl. 2): S56-S63. DOI: 10.1016/j.injury.2011.06.011

[31] Wang W, Yeung KWK. Bone grafts and biomaterials substitutes for bone defect repair: A review. Bioactive Materials. 2017;**2**(4):224-247

[32] Kinik H, Kalem M. Ilizarov segmental bone transport of infected

tibial nonunions requiring extensive debridement with an average distraction length of 9,5 centimetres. Is it safe? Injury. 2021;**52**(8):2425-2433

[33] Giannoudis PV, Faour O, Goff T, Kanakaris N, Dimitriou R. Masquelet technique for the treatment of bone defects: Tips-tricks and future directions. Injury. 2011;**42**(6):591-598

[34] Hertel R, Gerber A, Schlegel U, Cordey J, Rüegsegger P, Rahn BA. 10. Cancellous bone graft for skeletal reconstruction muscular versus periosteal bed — Preliminary report. Injury. 1994;**25**:SA59-SA70

[35] Perry CR. Bone repair techniques, bone graft, and bone graft substitutes. Clinical Orthopaedics and Related Research. 1999;**360**:71-86

[36] Jones AL, Bucholz RW, Bosse MJ, Mirza SK, Lyon TR, Webb LX, et al. Recombinant human BMP-2 and allograft compared with autogenous bone graft for reconstruction of Diaphyseal Tibial fractures with cortical defects. Journal of Bone and Joint Surgery. 2006;**88**(7):1431-1441

[37] Sarkar MR, Augat P, Shefelbine SJ, Schorlemmer S, Huber-Lang M, Claes L, et al. Bone formation in a long bone defect model using a platelet-rich plasma-loaded collagen scaffold. Biomaterials. 2006;**27**(9):1817-1823

[38] Ono I, Tateshita T, Satou M, Sasaki T, Matsumoto M, Kodama N. Treatment of large complex cranial bone defects by using hydroxyapatite ceramic implants. Plastic and Reconstructive Surgery. 1999;**104**(2):339-349

[39] Iwatsu J, Watanuki M, Yoshida S, Hitachi S, Watanabe M, Aizawa T. Clinical outcome of porous hydroxyapatite/collagen graft on bone defects following curettage of bone tumors. Journal of Biomedical Materials Research Part B Applied Biomaterials. 2022;**110**(10):2211-2216

[40] Qiu X, Chen Y, Qi X, Shi H, Wang J, Xiong J. Outcomes of cement beads and cement spacers in the treatment of bone defects associated with post-traumatic osteomyelitis. BMC Musculoskeletal Disorders. 2017;**18**(1):256

[41] Yao Q, Liu H, Lin X, Ma L, Zheng X, Liu Y, et al. 3D interpenetrated graphene foam/58S bioactive glass scaffolds for electrical-stimulation-assisted differentiation of rabbit mesenchymal stem cells to enhance bone regeneration. Journal of Biomedical Nanotechnology. 2019;**15**(3):602-611

[42] Leppik L, Oliveira KMC, Bhavsar MB, Barker JH. Electrical stimulation in bone tissue engineering treatments. European Journal of Trauma and Emergency Surgery. 2020;**46**(2):231-244

[43] Meng S, Rouabhia M, Zhang Z. Electrical stimulation in tissue regeneration. In: Applied Biomedical Engineering. London, United Kingdom: InTech; 2011

[44] Palanisamy P, Alam M, Li S, Chow SKH, Zheng Y. Low-intensity pulsed ultrasound stimulation for bone fractures healing. Journal of Ultrasound in Medicine. 2022;**41**(3):547-563

[45] Harrison A, Alt V. Low-intensity pulsed ultrasound (LIPUS) for stimulation of bone healing – A narrative review. Injury. 2021;**52**:S91-S96

[46] Shimizu T, Fujita N, Tsuji-Tamura K, Kitagawa Y, Fujisawa T, Tamura M, et al. Osteocytes as main responders to low-intensity pulsed ultrasound treatment during fracture healing. Scientific Reports. 2021;**11**(1):10298

[47] Walewicz K, Taradaj J, Rajfur K, Ptaszkowski K, Kuszewski MT, Sopel M, et al. The effectiveness of radial extracorporeal shock wave therapy In patients with chronic low Back pain: A prospective, randomized, single-blinded pilot study. Clinical Interventions in Aging. 2019;**14**:1859-1869

[48] Yao G, Chen J, Duan Y, Chen X. Efficacy of extracorporeal shock wave therapy for lateral epicondylitis: A systematic review and meta-analysis. BioMed Research International. 2020;**2020**:1-8

[49] Liao C-D, Xie G-M, Tsauo J-Y, Chen H-C, Liou T-H. Efficacy of extracorporeal shock wave therapy for knee tendinopathies and other soft tissue disorders: A meta-analysis of randomized controlled trials. BMC Musculoskeletal Disorders. 2018;**19**(1):278

[50] Liu T, Shindel AW, Lin G, Lue TF. Cellular signaling pathways modulated by low-intensity extracorporeal shock wave therapy. International Journal of Impotence Research. 2019;**31**(3):170-176

[51] Liu Y, Yushan M, Liu Z, Liu J, Ma C, Yusufu A. Complications of bone transport technique using the Ilizarov method in the lower extremity: A retrospective analysis of 282 consecutive cases over 10 years. BMC Musculoskeletal Disorders. 2020;**21**(1):354

[52] Aktuglu K, Erol K, Vahabi A. Ilizarov bone transport and treatment of critical-sized tibial bone defects: A narrative review. Journal of Orthopaedics and Traumatology. 2019;**20**(1):22

[53] Wang W, Yang J, Wang Y, Han G, Jia J-P, Xu M, et al. Bone transport using the Ilizarov method for osteosarcoma patients with tumor resection and neoadjuvant chemotherapy. Journal of Bone Oncology. 2019;**16**:100224, 1-8

[54] Verboket RD, Leiblein M, Janko M, Schaible A, Brune JC, Schröder K, et al. From two stages to one: Acceleration of the induced membrane (Masquelet) technique using human acellular dermis for the treatment of non-infectious large bone defects. European Journal of Trauma and Emergency Surgery. 2020;**46**(2):317-327

[55] Careri S, Vitiello R, Oliva MS, Ziranu A, Maccauro G, CP. Masquelet technique and osteomyelitis: Innovations and literature review. European Review for Medical and Pharmacological Sciences. 2019;**23**(2):210-216

[56] Ozaki H, Hamai R, Shiwaku Y, Sakai S, Tsuchiya K, Suzuki O. Mutual chemical effect of autograft and octacalcium phosphate implantation on enhancing intramembranous bone regeneration. Science and Technology of Advanced Materials. 2021;**22**(1):345-362

[57] DeBaun MR, Stahl AM, Daoud AI, Pan C, Bishop JA, Gardner MJ, et al. Preclinical induced membrane model to evaluate synthetic implants for healing critical bone defects without autograft. Journal of Orthopaedic Research. 2019;**37**(1):60-68

[58] Baldwin P, Li DJ, Auston DA, Mir HS, Yoon RS, Koval KJ. Autograft, allograft, and bone graft substitutes: Clinical evidence and indications for use in the setting of Orthopaedic trauma surgery. Journal of Orthopaedic Trauma. 2019;**33**(4):203-213

[59] Valtanen RS, Yang YP, Gurtner GC, Maloney WJ, Lowenberg DW. Synthetic and bone tissue engineering graft substitutes: What is the future? Injury. 2021;**52**:S72-S77. DOI: 10.1016/j.injury.2020.07.040

[60] Fernandez, de Grado G, Keller L, Idoux-Gillet Y, Wagner Q,

Musset AM, Benkirane-Jessel N, et al. Bone substitutes: A review of their characteristics, clinical use, and perspectives for large bone defects management. Journal of Tissue Engineering. 2018;**9**:1-18

[61] Bal Z, Kushioka J, Kodama J, Kaito T, Yoshikawa H, Korkusuz P, et al. BMP and TGFβ use and release in bone regeneration. Turkish Journal of Medical Sciences. 2020;**50**(7):1707-1722

[62] Zhao X, Han Y, Li J, Cai B, Gao H, Feng W, et al. BMP-2 immobilized PLGA/hydroxyapatite fibrous scaffold via polydopamine stimulates osteoblast growth. Materials Science and Engineering: C. 2017;**78**:658-666. DOI: 10.1016/j.msec.2017.03.186

[63] Wei Y, Zhu G, Zhao Z, Yin C, Zhao Q, Xu H, et al. Individualized plasticity autograft mimic with efficient bioactivity inducing osteogenesis. International Journal of Oral Science. 2021;**13**(1):14

[64] Zhang P, Han F, Li Y, Chen J, Chen T, Zhi Y, et al. Local delivery of controlled-release simvastatin to improve the biocompatibility of polyethylene terephthalate artificial ligaments for reconstruction of the anterior cruciate ligament. International Journal of Nanomedicine. 2016;**11**:465-478

[65] Ghorbani F, Ghalandari B, Sahranavard M, Zamanian A, Collins MN. Tuning the biomimetic behavior of hybrid scaffolds for bone tissue engineering through surface modifications and drug immobilization. Materials Science and Engineering: C. 2021;**130**(August):112434

[66] Rezaei H, Shahrezaee M, Jalali Monfared M, Fathi Karkan S, Ghafelehbashi R. Simvastatin-loaded graphene oxide embedded in polycaprolactone-polyurethane nanofibers for bone tissue engineering applications. Journal of Polymer Engineering. 2021;**41**(5):375-386

[67] Shahrezaie M, Moshiri A, Shekarchi B, Oryan A, Maffulli N, Parvizi J. Effectiveness of tissue engineered three-dimensional bioactive graft on bone healing and regeneration: An in vivo study with significant clinical value. Journal of Tissue Engineering and Regenerative Medicine. 2018;**12**(4):936-960

[68] Feng C, Xiao L, Yu JC, Li DY, Tang TY, Liao W, et al. Simvastatin promotes osteogenic differentiation of mesenchymal stem cells in rat model of osteoporosis through BMP-2/Smads signaling pathway. European Review for Medical and Pharmacological Sciences. 2020;**24**(1):434-443

[69] Shahrezaee M, Oryan A, Bastami F, Hosseinpour S, Shahrezaee MH, Kamali A. Comparative impact of systemic delivery of atorvastatin, simvastatin, and lovastatin on bone mineral density of the ovariectomized rats. Endocrine. 2018;**60**(1):138-150

[70] Leppik L, Zhihua H, Mobini S, Thottakkattumana Parameswaran V, Eischen-Loges M, Slavici A, et al. Combining electrical stimulation and tissue engineering to treat large bone defects in a rat model. Scientific Reports. 2018;**8**(1):1-14

[71] Zhang J, Liu Z, Tang J, Li Y, You Q, Yang J, et al. Fibroblast growth factor 2–induced human amniotic mesenchymal stem cells combined with autologous platelet rich plasma augmented tendon-to-bone healing. The Journal of Orthopaedic Translation. 2020;**24**:155-165

[72] Kao CT, Chen YJ, Huang TH, Lin YH, Hsu TT, Ho CC. Assessment of

the release profile of fibroblast growth factor-2-load mesoporous calcium silicate/poly-ε-caprolactone 3d scaffold for regulate bone regeneration. PRO. 2020;**8**(10):1-16

[73] Han L, Fang W-L, Jin B, Xu S-C, Zheng X, Hu Y-G. Enhancement of tendon-bone healing after rotator cuff injuries using combined therapy with mesenchymal stem cells and platelet rich plasma. European Review for Medical and Pharmacological Sciences. 2019;**23**:9075-9084

[74] Xie H, Cao L, Ye L, Du J, Shan G, Hu J, et al. Autogenous bone particles combined with platelet-rich plasma can stimulate bone regeneration in rabbits. Experimental and Therapeutic Medicine. 2020;**20**(6):1-1

[75] Liebig BE, Kisiday JD, Bahney CS, Ehrhart NP, Goodrich LR. The platelet-rich plasma and mesenchymal stem cell milieu: A review of therapeutic effects on bone healing. Journal of Orthopaedic Research. 2020;**38**(12):2539-2550

[76] Bao D, Sun J, Gong M, Shi J, Qin B, Deng K, et al. Combination of graphene oxide and platelet-rich plasma improves tendon–bone healing in a rabbit model of supraspinatus tendon reconstruction. Regenerative Biomaterials. 2021;**8**(6):rbab045

[77] Ghaffarpasand F, Shahrezaei M, Dehghankhalili M. Effects of platelet rich plasma on healing rate of long bone non-union fractures: A randomized double-blind placebo controlled clinical trial. Bull Emerg Trauma. 2016;**4**(3):134-140

[78] Qi Z, Xia P, Pan S, Zheng S, Fu C, Chang Y, et al. Combined treatment with electrical stimulation and insulin-like growth factor-1 promotes bone regeneration in vitro. PLoS One. 2018;**13**(5):e0197006

[79] Zhang X, Xing H, Qi F, Liu H, Gao L, Wang X. Local delivery of insulin/IGF-1 for bone regeneration: Carriers, strategies, and effects. Nano. 2020;**4**(4):242-255

[80] Teng C-F, Jeng L-B, Shyu W-C. Role of insulin-like growth factor 1 receptor signaling in stem cell Stemness and therapeutic efficacy. Cell Transplantation. 2018;**27**(9):1313-1319. DOI: 10.1177/0963689718779777

[81] Śmieszek A, Tomaszewski K, Kornicka K, Marycz K. Metformin promotes osteogenic differentiation of adipose-derived stromal cells and exerts pro-osteogenic effect stimulating bone regeneration. Journal of Clinical Medicine. 2018;**7**(12):482

[82] Shahrezaee M, Salehi M, Keshtkari S, Oryan A, Kamali A, Shekarchi B. In vitro and in vivo investigation of PLA/PCL scaffold coated with metformin-loaded gelatin nanocarriers in regeneration of critical-sized bone defects. Nanomedicine Nanotechnology, Biol Med. 2018;**14**(7):2061-2073. DOI: 10.1016/j.nano.2018.06.007

[83] Li Z, Wang H, Zhang K, Yang B, Xie X, Yang Z, et al. Bisphosphonate-based hydrogel mediates biomimetic negative feedback regulation of osteoclastic activity to promote bone regeneration. Bioactive Materials. 2022;**13**:9-22

[84] Qayoom I, Raina DB, Širka A, Tarasevičius Š, Tägil M, Kumar A, et al. Anabolic and antiresorptive actions of locally delivered bisphosphonates for bone repair. The Journal of Bone Joint Research. 2018;**7**(10):548-560. DOI: 10.1302/2046-3758.710.BJR-2018-0015.R2

[85] Sahranavard M, Sarkari S, Safavi S, Ghorbani F. Three-dimensional

bio-printing of decellularized extracellular matrix-based bio-inks for cartilage regeneration: A systematic review. Biomaterials Translational. 2022;**3**(2):105-115

[86] Kabirian F, Mozafari M. Decellularized ECM-derived bioinks: Prospects for the future. Methods. 2020;**171**(April):108-118

[87] Zhang X, Liu Y, Luo C, Zhai C, Li Z, Zhang Y, et al. Crosslinker-free silk/decellularized extracellular matrix porous bioink for 3D bioprinting-based cartilage tissue engineering. Materials Science and Engineering: C. 2020;**2021**(118):111388

[88] Park W, Gao G, Cho DW. Tissue-specific decellularized extracellular matrix bioinks for musculoskeletal tissue regeneration and modeling using 3d bioprinting technology. International Journal of Molecular Sciences. 2021;**22**(15):7837

[89] Lee H, Yang GH, Kim M, Lee JY, Huh JT, Kim GH. Fabrication of micro/nanoporous collagen/dECM/silk-fibroin biocomposite scaffolds using a low temperature 3D printing process for bone tissue regeneration. Materials Science and Engineering: C. 2017;**2018**(84):140-147

[90] Kim YS, Majid M, Melchiorri AJ, Mikos AG. Applications of decellularized extracellular matrix in bone and cartilage tissue engineering. Bioengineering & Translational Medicine. 2019;**4**(1):83-95

[91] Subramaniam S, Fang YH, Sivasubramanian S, Lin FH, Lin C-P. Hydroxyapatite-calcium sulfate-hyaluronic acid composite encapsulated with collagenase as bone substitute for alveolar bone regeneration. Biomaterials. 2016;**74**:99-108. DOI: 10.1016/j.biomaterials.2015.09.044

[92] Bendtsen ST, Quinnell SP, Wei M. Development of a novel alginate-polyvinyl alcohol-hydroxyapatite hydrogel for 3D bioprinting bone tissue engineered scaffolds. Journal of Biomedical Materials Research Part A. 2017;**105**(5):1457-1468

[93] Lee JB, Kim JE, Bae MS, Park SA, Balikov DA, Sung HJ, et al. Development of poly(ε-Caprolactone) scaffold loaded with simvastatin and beta-cyclodextrin modified hydroxyapatite inclusion complex for bone tissue engineering. Polymers (Basel). 2016;**8**(2):1-10

[94] Ghorbani F, Zamanian A, Behnamghader A, Jouparí MD. Microwave-induced rapid formation of biomimetic hydroxyapatite coating on gelatin-siloxane hybrid microspheres in 10X-SBF solution. E-Polymers. 2018;**18**(3):247-255

[95] Dewi Ana A, Ika HD. The use of hydroxyapatite bone substitute grafting for alveolar ridge preservation, sinus augmentation, and periodontal bone defect: A systematic review. Heliyon. 2018;**4**(10):e00884

[96] Walsh DP, Raftery RM, Chen G, Heise A, Fergal J. Rapid healing of a critical-sized bone defect using a collagen-hydroxyapatite scaffold to facilitate low dose, combinatorial growth factor delivery running title: Rapid bone tissue regeneration using a dual protein loaded collagen scaffold. Journal of Tissue Engineering and Regenerative Medicine. 2019;**13**(10):1843-1853

[97] Lodoso-Torrecilla I, van den Beucken JJJP, Jansen JA. Calcium phosphate cements: Optimization toward biodegradability. Acta Biomaterialia. 2021;**119**:1-12

[98] Yousefi A. A review of calcium phosphate cements and acrylic bone cements as injectable materials for bone

repair and implant fixation. The Journal of Applied Biomaterials & Functional Materials. 2019;**17**(4):1-21

[99] Wang J, Yin Q, Sanjun G, Yongwei W, Rui Y. Induced membrane technique in the treatment of infectious bone defect: A clinical analysis. Orthopaedics & Traumatology, Surgery & Research. 2019;**105**(3):535-539

[100] Jia C, Wang X, Yu S, Wu H, Shen J, Huang Q, et al. An antibiotic cement-coated locking plate as a temporary fixation for treatment of infected bone defects: A new method of stabilization. Journal of Orthopaedic Surgery and Research. 2020;**2**:1-8

[101] Brueckner T, Heilig P, Jordan MC, Paul MM, Blunk T, Meffert RH, et al. Biomechanical evaluation of promising different bone substitutes in a clinically relevant test set-up. Materials (Basel). 2019;**12**:1364

[102] Combal A, Thuau F, Fouasson-Chailloux A, Arrigoni P-P, Baud'huin M, Duteille F, et al. Preliminary results of the "Capasquelet" technique for managing femoral bone defects—Combining a Masquelet induced membrane and Capanna vascularized fibula with an allograft. Journal of Personalized Medicine. 2021;**11**(8):774

[103] Langenbach F, Handschel J. Effects of dexamethasone, ascorbic acid and β-glycerophosphate on the osteogenic differentiation of stem cells in vitro. Stem cell reserach Ther. 2013;**4**(5):117. DOI: 10.1089/ten.teb.2011.0199

[104] Ho-Shui-Ling A, Bolander J, Rustom LE, Johnson AW, Luyten FPPC. Bone regeneration strategies: Engineered scaffolds, bioactive molecules and stem cells current stage and future perspectives. Biomaterials. 2018;**180**:143-162

[105] Trivedi S, Srivastava K, Gupta A, Saluja TS, Kumar S, Mehrotra D, et al. A quantitative method to determine osteogenic differentiation aptness of scaffold. Journal of Oral Biology and Craniofacial Research. 2020;**10**(2):158-160

[106] Lin H, Sohn J, Shen H, Langhans MTTR. Bone marrow mesenchymal stem cells: Aging and tissue engineering applications to enhance bone healing. Biomaterials. 2019;**203**:96-110

[107] Liu Y, Kuang B, Rothrauff BB, Tuan RS, Lin H. Robust bone regeneration through endochondral ossification of human mesenchymal stem cells within their own extracellular matrix. Biomaterials. 2019;**218**:119336

[108] Yuan-Zhe Jin JHL. Mesenchymal stem cell therapy for bone regeneration. Clinics in Orthopedic Surgery. 2018;**10**(3):271-278

[109] Sharma S, Sudhakara P, Singh J, Ilyas RA, Asyraf MRM, Razman MR. Critical review of biodegradable and bioactive polymer composites for bone tissue engineering and drug delivery applications. Polymers (Basel). 2021;**13**(16):2623

[110] Ghorbani F, Zamanian A. An efficient functionalization of dexamethasone-loaded polymeric scaffold with [3-(2,3-epoxypropoxy)-propyl]-trimethoxysilane coupling agent for bone regeneration: Synthesis, characterization, and in vitro evaluation. Journal of Bioactive and Compatible Polymers. 2020;**35**(2):139-159

[111] Ghorbani F, Ghalandari B, Khan AL, Li D, Zamanian A, Yu B. Decoration of electrical conductive

polyurethane-polyaniline/polyvinyl alcohol matrixes with mussel-inspired polydopamine for bone tissue engineering. Biotechnology Progress. 2020;**36**(6):e3043

[112] Öfkeli F, Demir D, Bölgen N. Biomimetic mineralization of chitosan/gelatin cryogels and in vivo biocompatibility assessments for bone tissue engineering. Journal of Applied Polymer Science. 2021;**138**(14):1-12

[113] Sarparast Z, Abdoli R, Rahbari A, Varmazyar M, Kashyzadeh KR. Experimental and numerical analysis of permeability in porous media. International Journal of Engineering, Transactions B: Applications. 2020;**33**(11):2408-2415

[114] Madhumathi K, Binulal NS, Nagahama H, Tamura H, Shalumon KT, Selvamurugan N, et al. Preparation and characterization of novel β-chitin-hydroxyapatite composite membranes for tissue engineering applications. International Journal of Biological Macromolecules. 2009;**44**(1):1-5

[115] Li J, Chen M, Fan X, Zhou H. Recent advances in bioprinting techniques: Approaches, applications and future prospects. Journal of Translational Medicine. 2016;**14**(1):271

[116] Miao S, Zhu W, Castro NJ, Leng J, Zhang LG. Four-dimensional printing hierarchy scaffolds with highly biocompatible smart polymers for tissue engineering applications. Tissue Engineering Part C: Methods. 2016;**22**(10):952-963

[117] Tang G, Zhang H, Zhao Y, Li X, Yuan X, Wang M. Prolonged release from PLGA/HAp scaffolds containing drug-loaded PLGA/gelatin composite microspheres. Journal of Materials Science. Materials in Medicine. 2012;**23**(2):419-429

[118] Hidalgo Pitaluga L, Trevelin Souza M, Dutra Zanotto E, Santocildes Romero M, Hatton P. Electrospun F18 bioactive glass/PCL—Poly (ε-caprolactone)—Membrane for guided tissue regeneration. Materials (Basel). 2018;**11**(3):400

[119] Sahebalzamani M, Ziminska M, McCarthy HO, Levingstone TJ, Dunne NJ, Hamilton AR. Advancing bone tissue engineering one layer at a time: A layer-by-layer assembly approach to 3D bone scaffold materials. Biomaterials Science. 2022;**10**(11):2734-2758

[120] Abbasi N, Hamlet S, Love RM, Nguyen N. Porous scaffolds for bone regeneration. Journal of Science: Advanced Materials and Devices. 2020;**5**(1):1-9. DOI: 10.1016/j.jsamd.2020.01.007

[121] Ranjbari E, Bazgir S, Shirazi MMA. Needleless electrospinning of poly(acrylic acid) superabsorbent: Fabrication, characterization and swelling behavior. Polymer Testing. 2020;**84**:106403. DOI: 10.1016/j.polymertesting.2020.106403

[122] Takaku T, Hattori Y, Sasaki T, Sakamoto T, Otsuka M. Evaluation of swelling properties and drug release from mechanochemical pre-gelatinized glutinous rice starch matrix tablets by near infrared spectroscopy. Journal of Near Infrared Spectroscopy. 2021;**29**(2):92-101

[123] Koc FE, Altıncekic TG. Investigation of gelatin/chitosan as potential biodegradable polymer films on swelling behavior and methylene blue release kinetics. Polymer Bulletin. 2020;**78**:3383-3398. DOI: 10.1007/s00289-020-03280-7

[124] Nokoorani YD, Shamloo A. Comparison of the effect of EDC and glutaraldehyde as cross-linkers on morphology and swelling ratio of gelatin/chitosan scaffolds for use in skin tissue engineering. In: 25th National and 3rd International Iranian Conference on Biomedical Engineering (ICBME), Qom, Iran. 2018. pp. 1-4. DOI: 10.1109/ICBME.2018.8703585

[125] Saarai A, Kasparkova V, Sedlacek T, Saha P. On the development and characterisation of crosslinked sodium alginate/gelatine hydrogels. Journal of the Mechanical Behavior of Biomedical Materials. 2013;**18**:152-166. DOI: 10.1016/j.jmbbm.2012.11.010

[126] Mohamed MM. Preparation of PVA/Bioactive Glass Nanocomposite Scaffolds. In Vitro Studies for Applications as Biomaterials. Association with Active Molecules [Thesis]. Egypt: University of Cairo; 2013

[127] Yuan L, Wu Y, Gu Q, sheng, El-Hamshary H, El-Newehy M, Mo X. Injectable photo crosslinked enhanced double-network hydrogels from modified sodium alginate and gelatin. International Journal of Biological Macromolecules. 2017;**96**:569-577

[128] Eltom A, Zhong G, Muhammad A. Scaffold techniques and designs in tissue engineering functions and purposes: A review. Advances in Materials Science and Engineering. 2019;**2019**:1-13

[129] Mabrouk M, Beherei HH, Das DB. Recent progress in the fabrication techniques of 3D scaffolds for tissue engineering. Materials Science & Engineering. C, Materials for Biological Applications. 2020;**110**:1-33

[130] Collins MN, Ren G, Young K, Pina S, Reis RL, Oliveira JM. Scaffold fabrication technologies and structure/function properties in bone tissue engineering. Advanced Functional Materials. 2021;**31**(21):2010609

[131] Ghorbani F, Sahranavard M, Mousavi Nejad Z, Li D, Zamanian A, Yu B. Surface functionalization of three dimensional-printed polycaprolactone-bioactive glass scaffolds by grafting gelma under uv irradiation. Frontiers in Materials. 2020;**7**(December):1-17

[132] Khoshnood N, Shahrezayee MH, Shahrezayee M, Shams A, Zamanian A. Biological study of polyethyleneimine functionalized polycaprolactone 3D printed scaffolds for bone tissue engineering. Journal of Applied Polymer Science. 2022;**139**(29):e52628. DOI: 10.1002/app.52628

[133] Bernal PN, Delrot P, Loterie D, Li Y, Malda J, Moser C, et al. Volumetric bioprinting of complex living-tissue constructs within seconds. Advanced Materials. 2019;**31**(42):1904209

[134] Zhang L, Yang G, Johnson BN, Jia X. Three-dimensional (3D) printed scaffold and material selection for bone repair. Acta Biomaterialia. 2019;**84**(November):16-33

[135] Sahranavard M, Zamanian A, Ghorbani F, Shahrezaee MH. A critical review on three dimensional-printed chitosan hydrogels for development of tissue engineering. Bioprinting. 2020;**17**:e00063

[136] Choi YJ, Park H, Ha DH, Yun HS, Yi HG, Lee H. 3D bioprinting of in vitro models using hydrogel-based bioinks. Polymers (Basel). 2021;**13**(3):1-18

[137] Groll J, Burdick JA, Cho DW, Derby B, Gelinsky M, Heilshorn SC, et al. A definition of bioinks and their distinction from biomaterial inks. Biofabrication. 2019;**11**(1):013001

[138] Lee SJ, Esworthy T, Stake S, Miao S, Zuo YY, Harris BT, et al. Advances in 3D bioprinting for neural tissue engineering. Advanced Biosystems. 2018;**2**(4):1-18

[139] Gopinathan J, Noh I. Recent trends in bioinks for 3D printing. Biomaterials Research. 2018;**22**(1):11. DOI: 10.1186/s40824-018-0122-1

[140] Prina E, Mistry P, Sidney LE, Yang J, Wildman RD, Bertolin M, et al. 3D microfabricated scaffolds and microfluidic devices for ocular surface replacement: A review. Stem Cell Reviews and Reports. 2017;**13**(3):430-441. DOI: 10.1007/s12015-017-9740-6

[141] Bahraminasab M. Challenges on optimization of 3D-printed bone scaffolds. Biomedical Engineering Online. 2020;**19**(1):69. DOI: 10.1186/s12938-020-00810-2

[142] Blázquez-Carmona P, Sanz-Herrera JA, Martínez-Vázquez FJ, Domínguez J, Reina-Romo E. Structural optimization of 3D-printed patient-specific ceramic scaffolds for in vivo bone regeneration in load-bearing defects. Journal of the Mechanical Behavior of Biomedical Materials. 2021;**121**:104613

[143] Liang X, Gao J, Xu W, Wang X, Shen Y, Tang J, et al. Structural mechanics of 3D-printed poly(lactic acid) scaffolds with tetragonal, hexagonal and wheel-like designs. Biofabrication. 2019;**11**(3):035009. DOI: 10.1088/1758-5090/ab0f59

[144] Metz C, Duda GN, Checa S. Towards multi-dynamic mechano-biological optimization of 3D-printed scaffolds to foster bone regeneration. Acta Biomaterialia. 2020;**101**:117-127

[145] Pitacco P, Sadowska JM, O'Brien FJ, Kelly DJ. 3D bioprinting of cartilaginous templates for large bone defect healing. Acta Biomaterialia. 2022;**156**:61-74

[146] Sun X, Ma Z, Zhao X, Jin W, Zhang C, Ma J, et al. Three-dimensional bioprinting of multicell-laden scaffolds containing bone morphogenic protein-4 for promoting M2 macrophage polarization and accelerating bone defect repair in diabetes mellitus. Bioactive Materials. 2021;**6**(3):757-769

[147] Zhang J, Eyisoylu H, Qin X-H, Rubert M, Müller R. 3D bioprinting of graphene oxide-incorporated cell-laden bone mimicking scaffolds for promoting scaffold fidelity, osteogenic differentiation and mineralization. Acta Biomaterialia. 2021;**121**:637-652

[148] Dong L, Wang S-J, Zhao X-R, Zhu Y-F, Yu J-K. 3D- printed poly(ε-caprolactone) scaffold integrated with cell-laden chitosan hydrogels for bone tissue engineering. Scientific Reports. 2017;**7**(1):13412

[149] Khoshnood N, Shahrezaee MH, Shahrezaee M, Zamanian A. Three-dimensional bioprinting of tragacanth/hydroxyapaptite modified alginate bioinks for bone tissue engineering with tunable printability and bioactivity. Journal of Applied Polymer Science. 2022;**139**(36):e52833

[150] Hao Y, Wang L, Jiang W, Wu W, Ai S, Shen L, et al. 3D printing hip prostheses offer accurate reconstruction, stable fixation, and functional recovery for revision Total hip arthroplasty with complex acetabular bone defect. Engineering. 2020;**6**(11):1285-1290

[151] Wang W, Zhang B, Li M, Li J, Zhang C, Han Y, et al. 3D printing of PLA/n-HA composite scaffolds with customized mechanical properties and biological functions for bone tissue engineering. Composites. Part B, Engineering. 2021;**224**:109192

[152] Li JJ, Dunstan CR, Entezari A, Li Q, Steck R, Saifzadeh S, et al. A novel bone substitute with high bioactivity, strength, and porosity for repairing large and load-bearing bone defects. Advanced Healthcare Materials. 2019;**8**:e1801298

[153] Singh S, Choudhury D, Yu F, Mironov V, Naing MW. In situ bioprinting – Bioprinting from benchside to bedside? Acta Biomaterialia. 2020;**101**:14-25

[154] Cohen DL, Lipton JI, Bonassar LJ, Lipson H. Additive manufacturing for in situ repair of osteochondral defects. Biofabrication. 2010;**2**(3):035004

[155] Keriquel V, Guillemot F, Arnault I, Guillotin B, Miraux S, Amédée J, et al. In vivo bioprinting for computer- and robotic-assisted medical intervention: Preliminary study in mice. Biofabrication. 2010;**2**(1):014101

[156] Li L, Shi J, Ma K, Jin J, Wang P, Liang H, et al. Robotic in situ 3D bio-printing technology for repairing large segmental bone defects. Journal of Advanced Research. 2021;**30**:75-84

[157] Ye X, He J, Wang S, Han Q, You D, Feng B, et al. A hierarchical vascularized engineered bone inspired by intramembranous ossification for mandibular regeneration. International Journal of Oral Science. 2022;**14**(1):31

[158] Jia Y, Zhu Y, Qiu S, Xu J, Chai Y. Exosomes secreted by endothelial progenitor cells accelerate bone regeneration during distraction osteogenesis by stimulating angiogenesis. Stem Cell Research & Therapy. 2019;**10**:12

[159] Kérourédan O, Hakobyan D, Rémy M, Ziane S, Dusserre N, Fricain J-C, et al. In situ prevascularization designed by laser-assisted bioprinting: Effect on bone regeneration. Biofabrication. 2019;**11**(4):045002

[160] Kuss MA, Wu S, Wang Y, Untrauer JB, Li W, Lim JY, et al. Prevascularization of 3D printed bone scaffolds by bioactive hydrogels and cell co-culture. Journal of Biomedical Materials Research Part B: Applied Biomaterials. 2018;**106**(5):1788-1798

[161] Nulty J, Freeman FE, Browe DC, Burdis R, Ahern DP, Pitacco P, et al. 3D bioprinting of prevascularised implants for the repair of critically-sized bone defects. Acta Biomaterialia. 2021;**126**:154-169

[162] Lu W, Ding Z, Liu F, Shan W, Cheng C, Xu J, et al. Dopamine delays articular cartilage degradation in osteoarthritis by negative regulation of the NF-κB and JAK2/STAT3 signaling pathways. Biomedicine & Pharmacotherapy. 2019;**119**(May):109419. DOI: 10.1016/j.biopha.2019.109419

[163] Yang Z, Shi Y, Wei X, He J, Yang S, Dickson G, et al. Fabrication and repair of cartilage defects with a novel acellular cartilage matrix scaffold. Tissue Engineering Part C Methods. 2010;**16**(5):865-876

[164] Daly AC, Freeman FE, Gonzalez-Fernandez T, Critchley SE, Nulty J, Kelly DJ. 3D bioprinting for cartilage and Osteochondral tissue engineering. Advanced Healthcare Materials. 2017;**6**(22):1-20

[165] Bruyas A, Lou F, Stahl AM, Gardner M, Maloney W, Goodman S, et al. Systematic characterization of 3D-printed PCL/β-TCP scaffolds for biomedical devices and bone tissue engineering: Influence of composition and porosity. Journal of Materials Research. 2018;**33**(14):1948-1959

[166] Kilian D, Ahlfeld T, Akkineni AR, Bernhardt A, Gelinsky M, Lode A. 3D bioprinting of osteochondral tissue substitutes – in vitro-chondrogenesis in multi-layered mineralized constructs. Scientific Reports. 2020;**10**(1):8277

[167] Shim J-H, Jang K-M, Hahn SK, Park JY, Jung H, Oh K, et al. Three-dimensional bioprinting of multilayered constructs containing human mesenchymal stromal cells for osteochondral tissue regeneration in the rabbit knee joint. Biofabrication. 2016;**8**(1):014102

Chapter 2

Neonatal Fractures

Nikolaos Laliotis

Abstract

A neonatal fracture is a severe complication creating problems regarding diagnosis and appropriate management. Diagnosis from the neonatologist occasionally is difficult. A paediatric orthopaedic surgeon is required to evaluate the neonate, and confirm diagnosis and treatment. Clavicle fracture is the most common injury that must be differentiated occasionally from neonatal brachial plexus palsy. The clinical signs are crepitus, swelling, bony prominence, with the restriction of the movements of the arm. Occasionally, the fracture is diagnosed later. Clavicle pseudoarthrosis is a rare dysplasia. Fracture of the femur or the humerus presents with swelling, crepitus and deformity of the limb, creating difficulties in clothing, bathing and feeding. Most commonly are found in urgent caesarean delivery or complicated dystocia with overweighted neonates. Bone fragility diseases (osteogenesis imperfecta, hypophosphatasia, arthrogryposis) are diagnosed from neonatal fractures. Conservative treatment with immobilization is the method of choice. Extremely rare is surgical treatment. Premature and low-weighted babies are in high risk to sustain fractures. Epiphyseal fractures of the distal femoral or humeral epiphysis are rare fractures, difficult to be diagnosed initially. They require immediate reduction to avoid permanent lesion of the growth plate. Fractures of forearm, tibia or vertebrae are extremely rare and associated with a bone fragility disease.

Keywords: neonatal fracture, perinatal femoral fracture, perinatal humerus fracture, fragile neonate bone, premature and low weight neonates, birth related fractures

1. Introduction

Neonatal fractures are extremely rare. Initial diagnosis is occasionally obscure and clinical signs of oedema, crepitus, and mainly discomfort of the neonate are the main symptoms that the neonatologist is evaluating. The incidence of neonatal fractures is reported to be less than 1 per 1000 births. In a previous report among 158,035 full term neonates, fracture was demonstrated in 1174 of them (0.74%). In a recent survey in UK, in the period 2000–2016, in 87,461 live births, 66 sustained a fracture, with the clavicle fracture being the most common, as found in 46 cases. This is a low incidence overall of 0.075% [1, 2]. Increased fetus weight and vaginal delivery with associated labor dystocia were initially reported as predisposing factors. But several reports of fractures with cesarean delivery (CS) are reported as well. Preterm with small for gestational age babies are in increased risk for a neonatal fracture. Multiple birth, breech delivery, increased maternal body weight are among the risk factors for a neonatal fracture. Neonatal fractures may present as the initial sign of underlying bone fragility. Neonatal fractures are occasionally diagnosed in uncomplicated labor. A neonatal fracture may also be diagnosed after discharge from the maternity hospital, usually found from the callus formation or the persistent discomfort of the neonate [3–7].

2. Clavicle fractures

Fractures of the clavicle are the most common neonatal fractures. They are usually found in vaginal delivery of an overweight neonate. Shoulder dystocia is a severe complication during birth and immediate action is required from the obstetrician in order to avoid respiratory disturbance of the neonate. The fracture of the clavicle reduces the shoulder tension and promotes the early delivery of the neonate. Otherwise the hyperextension of the neck may lead to severe brachial plexus palsy. A fracture of the clavicle in a neonate can be diagnosed without history of dystocia, most commonly after a cesarean delivery. Urgent cesarean births have a higher incidence of clavicle fractures. Delayed deliveries over 39 weeks of gestation are reported with a higher incidence of clavicle fracture and brachial plexus palsy [8–14].

The main clinical sign is the restricted Moro reaction sign (Moro (startle) reflex, arms abduct in response to sensation of falling) that is the reduced abduction and external rotation of the affected arm. This is the most common examination test that the neonatologist performs in the newborn. The newborn has active movements of the wrist and fingers and easy flexion of the elbow in the affected side. The newborn expresses discomfort and is crying while changing clothes or while moving the arm while breast feeding. Oedema in the clavicle region appears usually in the 2nd and 3rd day, with crepitus while examining the clavicle. The clavicle ossifies following intramembranous and not endochondral ossification. It produces early an enlarged callus that is remodeled and the signs of the clavicle fracture are eliminated by the 3d month. Clinical signs are often obscure early and the family notices the presence of the enlarged callus in the clavicle region after a week time. There are normal movements of the affected side and even the Moro sign may have been reported as normal.

Radiological examination confirms the diagnosis and is mainly performed for the medico legal issues in case that there are associated lesions as brachial plexus palsy. Radiological examination is not always required since in typical cases we can reassure the parents for the benign course of the clavicle fracture. Ultrasound examination from an experienced radiologist can assist by confirming the disruption of the cortical continuity. There is no specific treatment that is required for this fracture. We inform the nurses and the family for the appropriate dressing and bathing of the neonate and to avoid the elevation of the affected arm. In a few days the neonate is moving the arm without discomfort. The arm is kept in the relaxed position with the elbow in 90 degrees of flexion, in the anterior part of the body (**Figures 1** and **2**).

The presence of an enlarged lump on the right clavicle of a baby, after several months, must be differentiated from congenital clavicle pseudoarthrosis. This is an extremely rare dysplasia, usually diagnosed in the preschool age, as it is a painless lump in the clavicle. Appropriate imaging with X-ray and CT scan confirms the diagnosis of the congenital pseudoarthrosis. There is absence of history of birth trauma. This dysplasia can be treated surgically with appropriate excision and plating, mainly for esthetic reasons. A new born with bilateral pseudoarthrosis of the clavicle that presented spontaneous recovery has been reported [15, 16] (**Figures 3** and **4**).

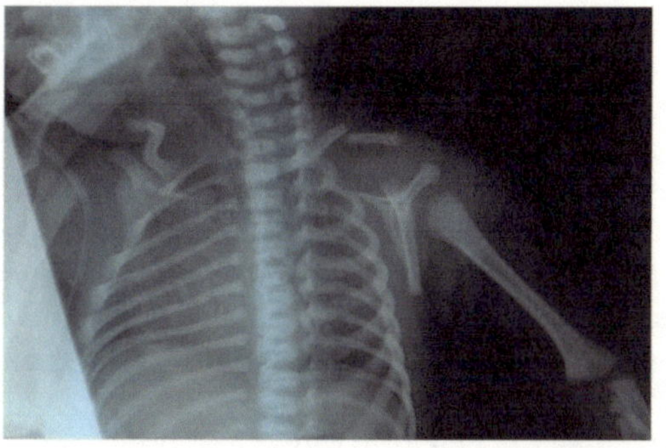

Figure 1.
Fracture of left clavicle.

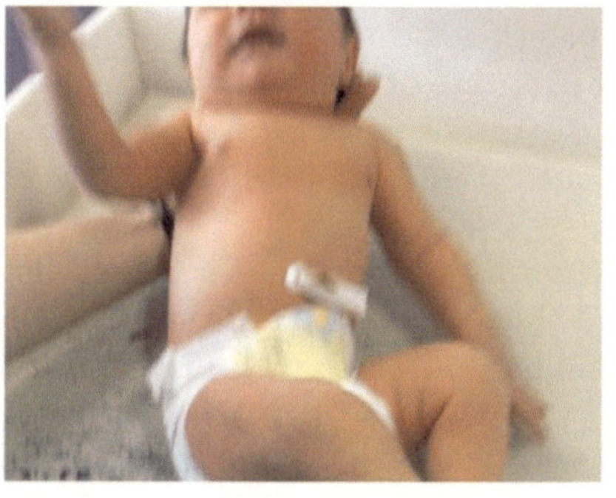

Figure 2.
Unable to perform the Moro reaction with the left arm.

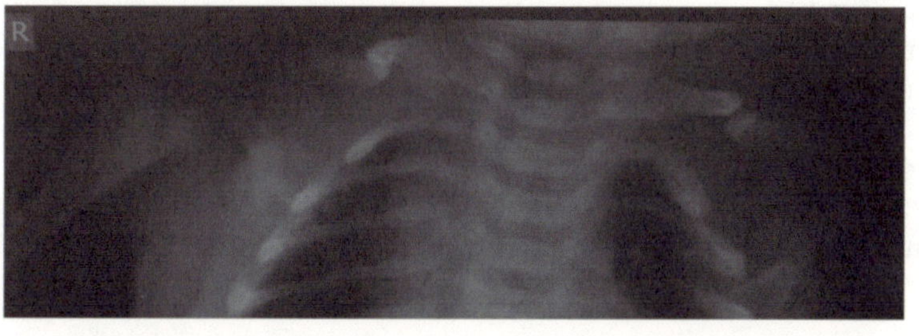

Figure 3.
X-ray-s of bilateral clavicle pseudoarthrosis with spontaneous union at a year time.

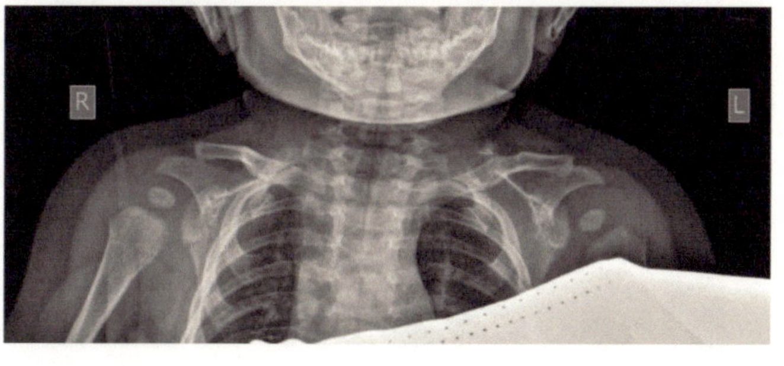

Figure 4.
X-ray-s of bilateral clavicle pseudoarthrosis with spontaneous union at a year time.

3. Neonatal femoral fractures

A neonatal femoral fracture is a rare but severe complication of the birth. The reported incidence is about 0.1/10000 births [17]. Although was believed that elective cesarean delivery would eliminate the incidence of birth trauma, this is not confirmed, and several reported neonatal femoral fractures are associated with CS. Femoral fracture in CS is an extremely rare complication. Urgent CS, increased birth weight, breech position, fibromatosis of the uterus, inadequate uterine relaxation, inadequate incision in the uterine segment are reported as predisposing factors for femoral fractures in CS [1–5, 17–21].

The obstetrician may feel the cracking sound and observe the pathological mobility of the femur, but this is uncommon. The examining pediatrician and the nurse will notice the swelling of the fractured femur and the abnormal shape and movements of the leg. The neonate is crying and dressing is extremely painful. Suspicion for the fractured femur may not be noticed until the 2nd and 3rd day of the life. Mother will report the permanent irritation of the neonate, the difficulties for breast feeding, since every movement causes crying. A case of a spiral femur fracture diagnosed 9 days postpartum, after an elective CS for the breech presentation has been reported [22].

Diagnosis is confirmed with appropriate X-ray examination. Fractures commonly affect the proximal third and the diaphysis of the femur. The proximal part is shifted in flexion and abduction, due to the imbalance of the muscle action (**Figures** 5 and **6**).

Treatment is provided with appropriate skin traction, either with Bryant's traction (both limbs suspended in the air vertically at 90°) or with simple skin traction. We use bilateral traction, with hips flexed in 90° and the buttock in a distance from the bed. We use simple skin traction in fractures in the middle third of the femur. Breast feeding becomes difficult, as the mother must lie in an uncomfortable position and the neonate is trying to feed by flexing the head, while it is in the traction. With patience and assistance from the nurse, this can be achieved. In premature children that must remain incubated or in the box, this traction is applied in their box [23, 24].

Fractures are united with excessive callus formation (**Figure** 7).

Usually a period of 2–3 weeks in traction is adequate to remove the traction. Use of Pavlik harness has also been recommended, with appropriate balance of the fractured

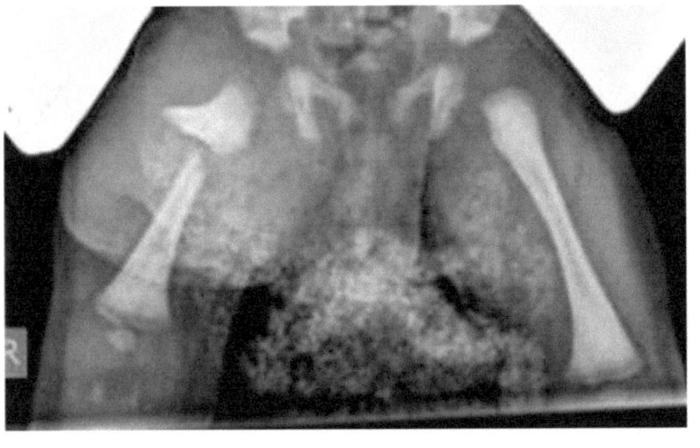

Figure 5.
The initial X-ray with a spiral fracture, with flexion and abduction of the proximal part.

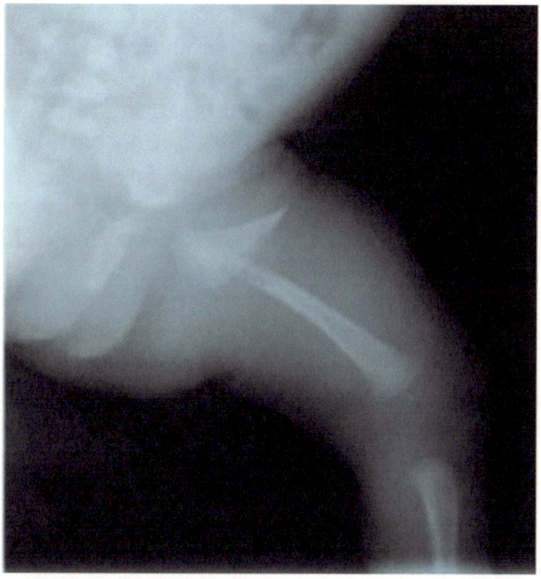

Figure 6.
Initial X-ray of the fractured femur with severe displacement in flexion and abduction of the proximal part. Treatment provided was skin traction with Bryant's method, for both legs.

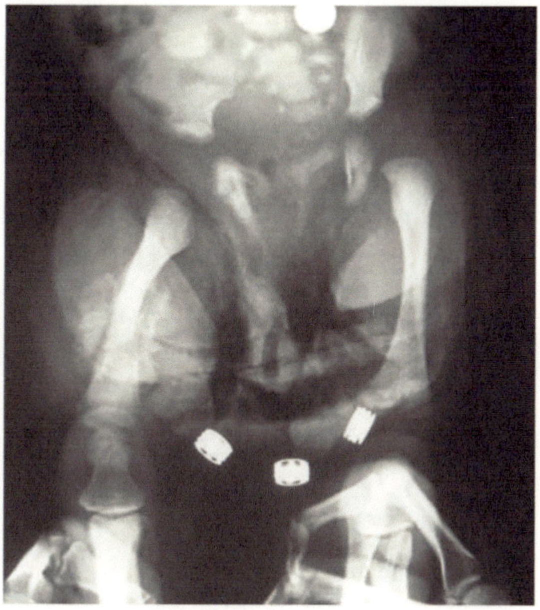

Figure 7.
Massive callus formation of the fractured right femur, in 2 months.

parts of the femur but is not a stable position mainly during the first week. Use of the harness requires frequent adjustments and the nursing stuff is unfamiliar with these corrections. We recommend the use of the harness after at least 10 days of traction, with caution, since the oversight of a pediatric orthopedic surgeon is of great importance in order to retain the appropriate reduction. Alternative methods of immobilization have been reported. Strapping the thigh to abdomen or the use of a hip spica are also described methods of immobilization [18]. We recommend for the neonate with a fractured femur the use of skin traction with Bryant's method as the safest and comfortable treatment. We have treated 5 neonates with femoral fractures, using skin traction over the past 20 years and we report very good results. We have not observed any rotational deviations and no leg length discrepancy in the first years of life.

The natural history is the early remodeling of the fracture. The child is observed up the age of 2–3 years old, to ensure the final leg length discrepancy and the appropriate shape of the femur. During the treatment period with skin traction it is of paramount importance to correct possible severe external rotation of the femur, since rotational deformities are not corrected with the remodeling process (**Figures 8** and **9**).

Surgical treatment is not recommended for the neonatal fracture. A case from Italy was reported using an external fixator for a neonate with lumbar myelomeningocele and fractured femur [25]. In case that fractured parts show severe angulations that must be corrected with appropriate change of the traction. We have treated an extremely rare case of a neonate that the fractured segment was caught under the skin. Despite the use of Bryant's traction and appropriate manipulation this was not corrected. We performed a minimal skin incision to reduce the fracture by splinting the muscles and stabilized temporally the segments with a K-wire and hip spica.

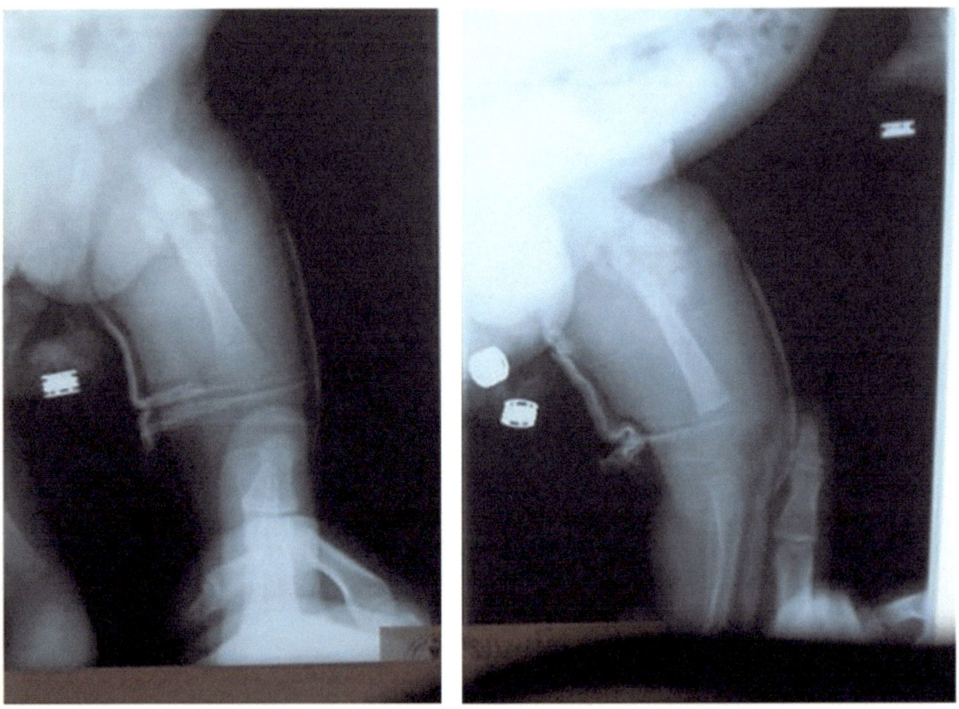

(a) (b)

Figure 8.
Excessive callus formation at 3 weeks of the fractured neonate femur.

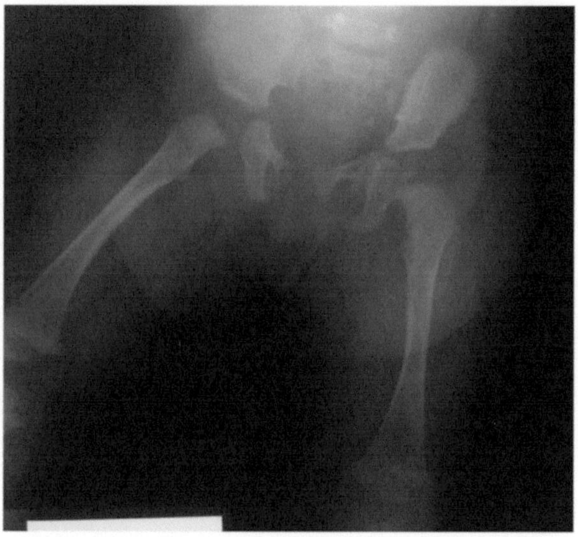

Figure 9.
At 1 year there is complete remodeling of the fractured left femur.

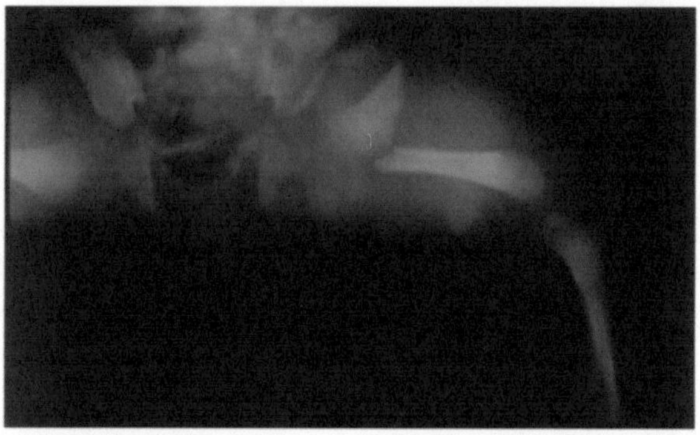

Figure 10.
Severe displacement and entrapment of the proximal part under the skin, despite use of Gallow's traction.

The neonate was closely observed with appropriate support from neonatologists. He had an uneventful recovery (**Figures 10** and **11**).

4. Fragility neonatal fractures

Fractured neonatal femur may be the initial sign of an underlying disease with bone fragility. Osteogenesis imperfecta (OI) is a heterogeneous connective tissue disorder characterized from severe osteoporosis. The synthesis of collagen type I is disrupted due to pathogenic genes. There is low bone mass with bone fragility that leads to recurrent fractures of the axial skeleton and the long bones resulting in severe deformities. Although there have been reported to be more than 20 types of gene

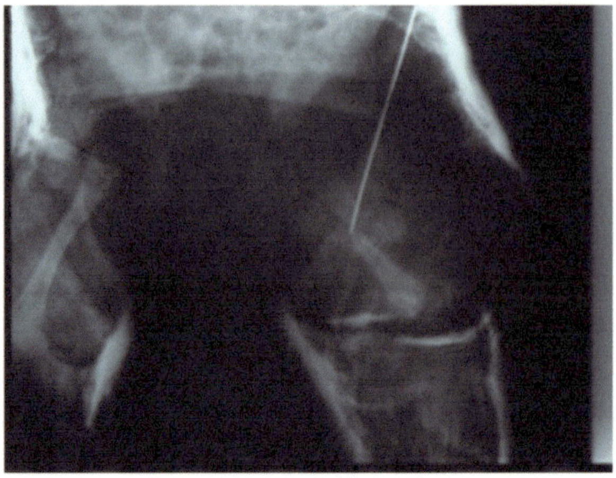

Figure 11.
Minimal incision, release of muscles and reduction, stabilized with a K-wire and hip spica. Apparent callus formation in a week time after reduction.

heterogeneity of OI, the clinical phenotype classification of Silence remains a valuable description of the severity of the disorder. The lethal form (type 2) presents with intrauterine fractures diagnosed with the prenatal ultrasonography. Long bones are described with bowing and shortening. X-ray examination in the neonate reveals several fractures, occasionally affecting the ribs as well. Femoral or tibial fractures are either spiral or transverse fractures. Type 3 OI presents with fractures without history of urgent manipulation of the neonate because of dystocia. On x-ray examination the bones are deformed and there is cortical thinning [26–28] (**Figure 12**).

With minor handling of the neonate, a crack may be felt and a new fracture may be diagnosed. There are clinical features with the prominent frontal bone, the short height of the neonate, and the ligamentous laxity. Child abuse must be ruled out in the presence of multiple fractures that are at different times of callus formation. Fractures found in clavicles, long bones or vertebrae are strong indications of the underlying

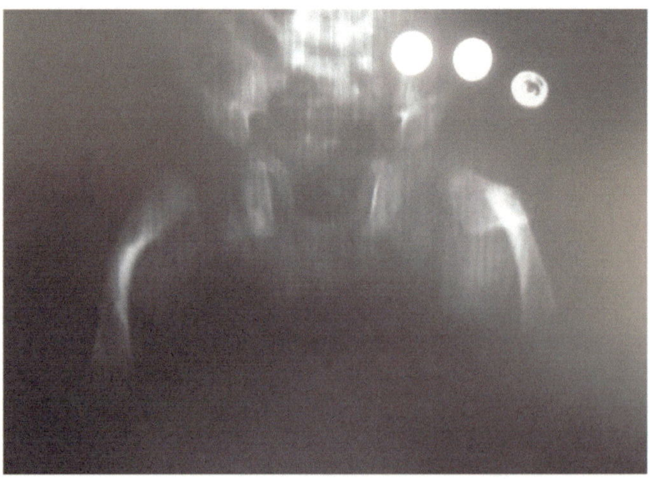

Figure 12.
Initial fracture of the left femur, following an uncomplicated normal vaginal delivery. Bowing and sclerosis of the right femur is noticed. The girl was diagnosed with osteogenesis imperfecta type 3.

bone fragility [29]. There are several metabolic diseases affecting the neonate that present with neonatal fractures. Disturbances of the calcium and phosphate metabolism as in phosphatasia and rickets are among the rare but severe diseases that are diagnosed through neonatal fractures, affecting both long bones and vertebrae and ribs. Appropriate laboratory investigations from neonatologists and endocrine pediatricians with genetic investigations, can provide an accurate diagnosis [30–34]. Treatment of neonatal fractures that are due to metabolic diseases follows the same principles as the femoral fractures of normal neonates with the use of Gallows traction. Modifications for use of traction in the neonatal box are described. Appropriate medical treatment is essential in order to reduce the number of fractures that may follow. Gene therapy is today the most promising treatment method for these severe forms. Stem cells therapy in the prenatal period has been reported [35].

Bilateral neonatal femoral fractures have been reported in a neonate with multiple congenital anomalies, with joint stiffness, similar to arthrogryposis. Arthrogryposis may be prenatally detected in a fetus with reduced mobility. It is important for the obstetrician to be informed of the joint stiffness in order to avoid vigorous movements that may lead to neonatal fractures [36] (**Figures 13** and **14**).

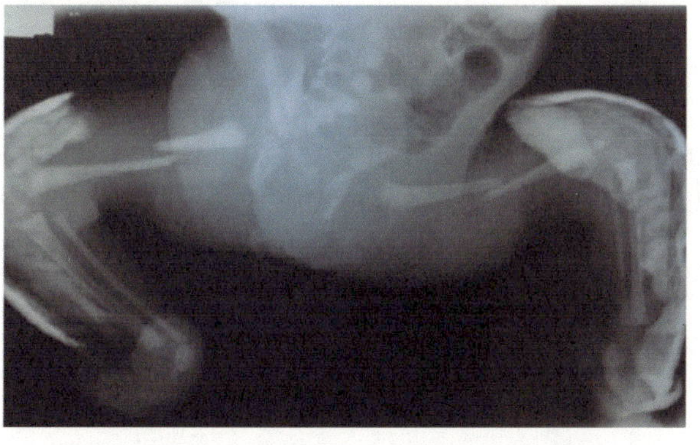

Figure 13.
Bilateral fractured femur in a neonate with complex stiff joints. Casts were applied for the club feet deformities. Treatment provided with Gallows traction. X-ray with united femoral fractures.

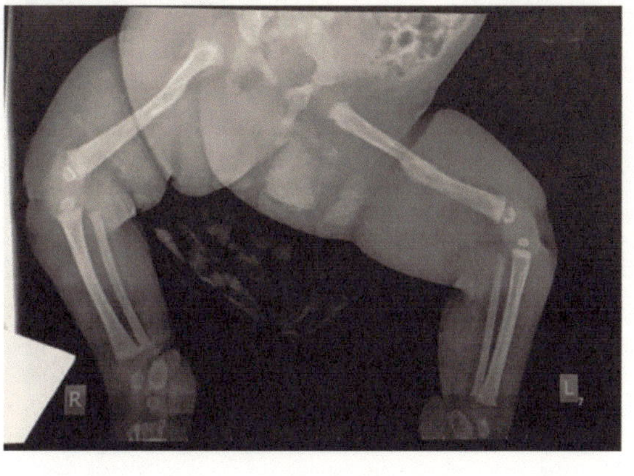

Figure 14.
Bilateral fractured femur in a neonate with complex stiff joints. Casts were applied for the club feet deformities. Treatment provided with Gallows traction. X-ray with united femoral fractures.

5. Metabolic bone disease in premature neonates

Premature neonates apart from the problems of low birth weight and respiratory disturbances, are associated with impaired mineralization of the bones. Several metabolic disturbances that include hypocalcemia, hypophosphatemia, and secondary hyperthyroidism must be ruled out in order to improve bone strength. Spontaneous fractures and deformities may appear and the nursing stuff and neonatologists must be very careful in the daily treatment of these premature neonates [37–42].

6. Distal femoral epiphysis lesion

A rare type of neonatal femoral fracture is the epiphysiolisthesis of the distal femoral epiphysis. The knee joint presents with effusion, there is limited movement of the affected limb, like a type of pseudoparalysis. The neonate is restless and bathing and dressing are difficult because of the reactions of the neonate. Diagnosis is obscure and septic arthritis of the neonate must be differentiated from epiphysiolisthesis. The distal femoral epiphysis ossification nucleus appears in infancy, but it is a small one and separation is not easily appearent on plain X-rays. Plain X-rays may appear with a minimal disruption of the metaphyseal corner. Ultrasound examination is helpful but cannot confirm diagnosis, as the fluid collection of the effusion may be a sign of infection. MRI examination will reveal the translation of the epiphysis. On MRI the hematoma is well demarcated with the separation of the epiphysis in the growth plate (**Figures 15–17**).

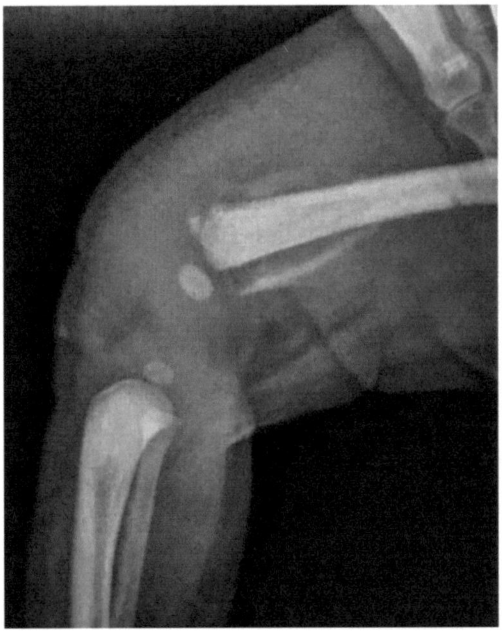

Figure 15.
Distal femoral epiphysiolisthesis Salter type 1, with calcification from the periosteal elevation. MRI demonstrates the hematoma and the periosteal elevation.

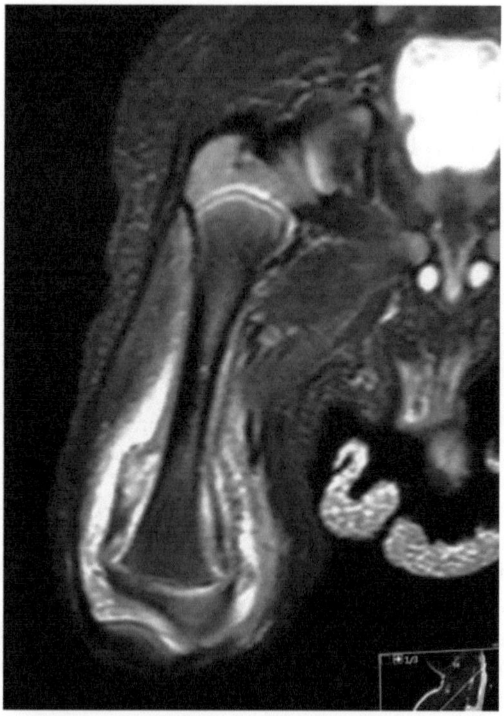

Figure 16.
Distal femoral epiphysiolisthesis Salter type 1, with calcification from the periosteal elevation. MRI demonstrates the hematoma and the periosteal elevation.

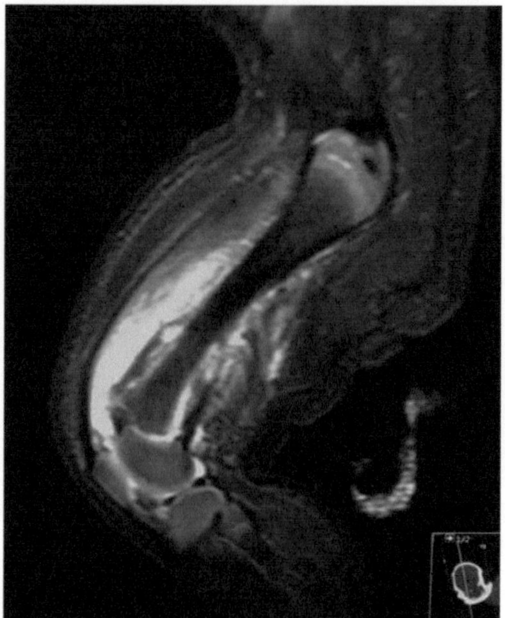

Figure 17.
Distal femoral epiphysiolisthesis Salter type 1, with calcification from the periosteal elevation. MRI demonstrates the hematoma and the periosteal elevation.

The distal femoral epiphysis is the most important for the proper growth of the limb, so the lesion must be diagnosed early in order to reduce the epiphysis. It is a Salter Harris type 1 or 2 lesion. The limb is immobilized in a light cast, incorporating the foot. If properly reduced, then growth of the limb may not be affected. The neonate must be followed for the next years to confirm the leg length equality. There have been reported cases with reduction and stabilization using K-wires. These injuries may create severe leg length discrepancy (LLD) and it is important for them to be evaluated by a pediatric orthopedic surgeon [43–48].

7. Humerus fractures

Fractures of the humerus are most commonly found in cases of urgent CS with the inappropriate handling of the fetus in an effort to complete the delivery and ensure proper respiration of the baby. Similar to femoral shaft fractures in the lower extremity, clinical signs are the absence of movement of the arm, angulations, oedema, and crepitus. Because of the decreased musculature of the humerus, this fracture is more easily diagnosed, as during bathing or dressing the neonate, the arm is angulating and the neonate is crying.

X-ray examination reveals the shaft fracture of the humerus (**Figures 18** and **19**). This must be differentiated from brachial plexus palsy with accurate clinical assessment. Occasionally radial nerve palsy may be found in conjunction with the neonate humerus fracture. Isolated radial nerve palsy has also been encountered in a neonate with a constriction from the umbilicus cord, without underlying fracture. It resolved gradually in a 3 weeks period [49–55] (**Figures 19** and **20**).

There are various methods for appropriate immobilization of the humerus fracture, but in case of a transverse fracture it is difficult to obtain a stable immobilization. Use of a U slab is uncomfortable and we prefer a Velpeau type of immobilization that is easily accepted and comfortable, enabling the proper breastfeeding of the neonate (**Figure 20**). It is important to achieve proper rotational alignment of the fracture since remodeling of the rotational deformities is poor. Excessive callus formation is found by the end of the 2nd week, and gradual mobilization is permitted. Humerus fractures may also present as the initial signs of metabolic disease and OI [29] (**Figure 21**).

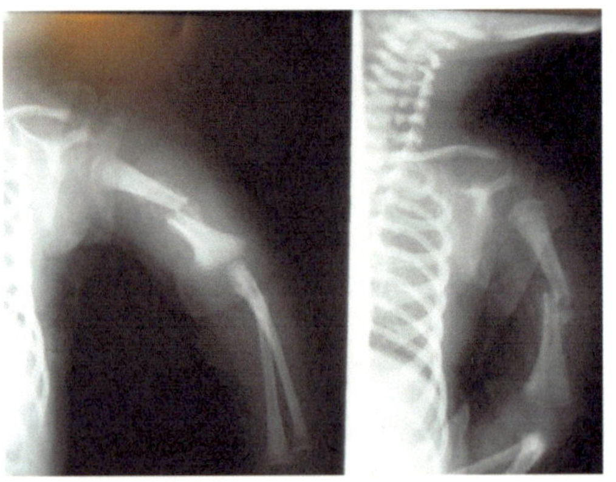

Figure 18.
Fracture of the left humerus after an emergency CS delivery.

DOI: http://dx.doi.org/10.5772/intechopen.110167

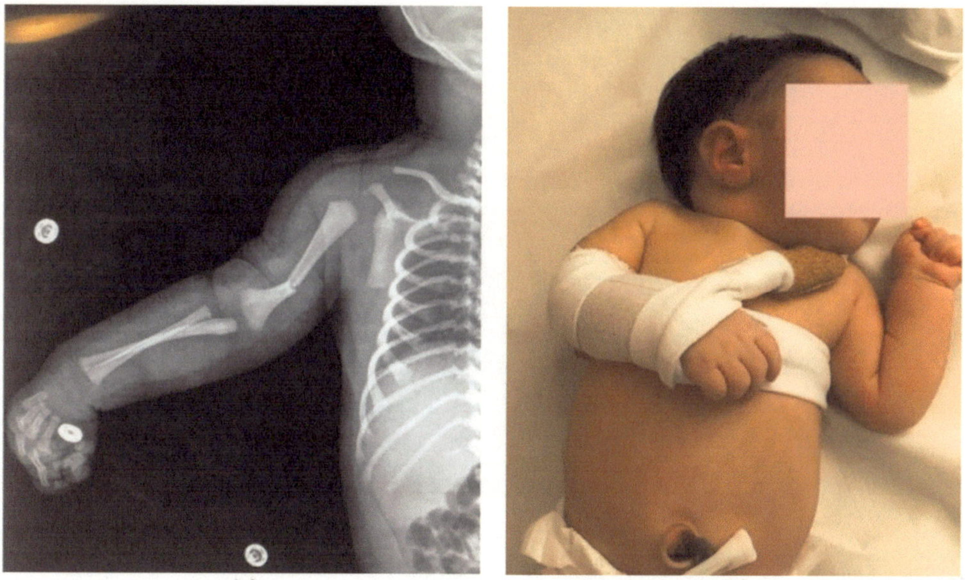

(a) (b)

Figure 19.
Fracture of the right humerus and treatment with appropriate strapping with Velpeau type of immobilization.

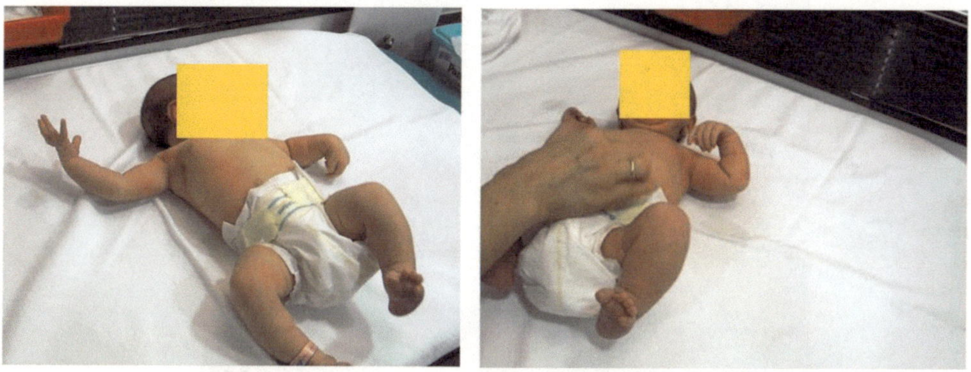

(a) (b)

Figure 20.
An isolated left radial nerve palsy. Note the flexion of the left elbow with the shoulder movement, while the wrist and fingers are not extending.

8. Fracture of the distal humerus epiphysis

An extremely rare injury is the epiphysiolisthesis of the distal humerus epiphysis that is commonly diagnosed with delay. Clinical signs are swelling of the elbow, with increased anxiety of the neonate and reduced mobility of the affected arm. The differential diagnosis includes neonatal septic arthritis and brachial plexus palsy. Appropriate clinical examination is essential for the correct diagnosis. Radiological examination reveals signs of possible elbow dislocation (**Figure 22**). There is malalignment of the humerus with the proximal part of the radius and ulna. The distal humerus epiphysis is not ossified and cannot be found separated from the metaphysic on X-ray. The medical

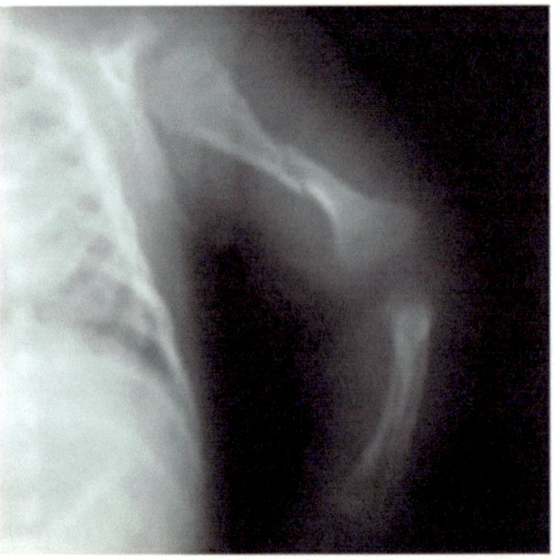

Figure 21.
Fracture left humerus, after a CS delivery, as the first sign of Osteogenesis imperfecta.

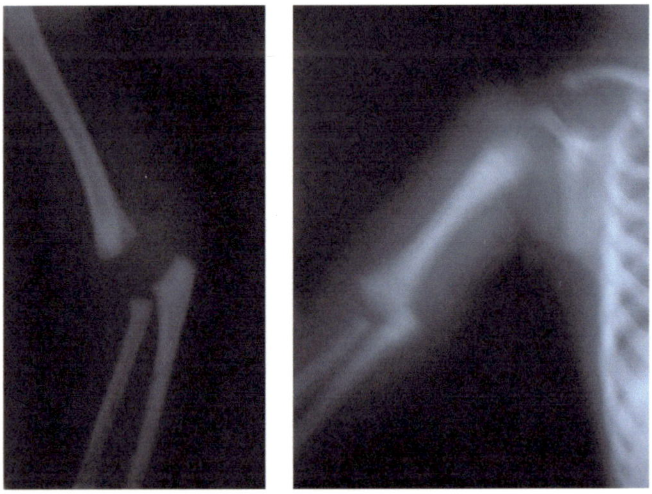

Figure 22.
Distal humerus epiphysiolisthesis appears on X-rays as an elbow dislocation.

history of possible forceful handling of the arm during delivery is of importance. Ultrasound examination is helpful by revealing the diffuse hematoma and the separation of the chondral epiphysis. MRI has been used in order to make the diagnosis. The distal epiphysis appears separated from the metaphysis of the humerus.

Appropriate reduction in the first 2–4 days is essential in order to restore the anatomy and appropriate elbow function. Reduction is easily performed in the first 1–2 days with an impressive resolution of the symptoms. The elbow becomes less swollen and the relief of the neonate appears almost immediately. Proper casting with a brace is important for a period of 2 weeks. Reduction must be performed under anesthesia, using C-arm and possibly with the addition of an arthrogram, in order to reassure the accurate reduction. Arthrogram in the neonate elbow is hard to be achieved with accuracy but in cases of a fracture with the hematoma of the joint that is swollen, it can be performed. Callus formation from the periosteal elevation in neonates is apparent early and reduction is not advised later than a period of a week.

K-wire stabilization is reported in cases of instability of the epiphysiolisthesis, but Salter type 1 and 2 are usually stable after appropriate reduction and cast immobilization is adequate. Remodeling of the humerus has been reported even in cases that the epiphysiolisthesis was diagnosed later and without reduction. But this extremely rare injury must be treated with adequate reduction in the initial first days [56–65].

9. Fractures of forearm

Fracture of the forearm is extremely rare and may be a sign of the underlying bone fragility, with similar fractures in the femur or humerus. Child abuse must be ruled out. Extremely rare is the report of a constriction band in the forearm with fracture of the underlying radius and ulna, with severe compromise of the vascularity of the forearm. Pseudorarthrosis of the radius or ulna as signs of neurofibromatosis are rarely diagnosed in the neonatal period. Hyperostosis of the forearm (Caffeys disease) is among the extremely rare cases with x-ray similar to neonatal fracture [66–70] (**Figures 23** and **24**).

10. Fractures of the tibia

These fractures are also extremely rare and are found in combination with fractures of the femur or humerus. Underlying bone fragility is suspected and investigations for possible OI or rickets must be performed. Neonate abuse syndrome must also be verified. We have followed a neonate that sustained fractures of the femur and tibia during birth after having a normal uncomplicated vaginal delivery. At the age of 2 years there is only short stature, without underlying metabolic disease (**Figures 25–27**).

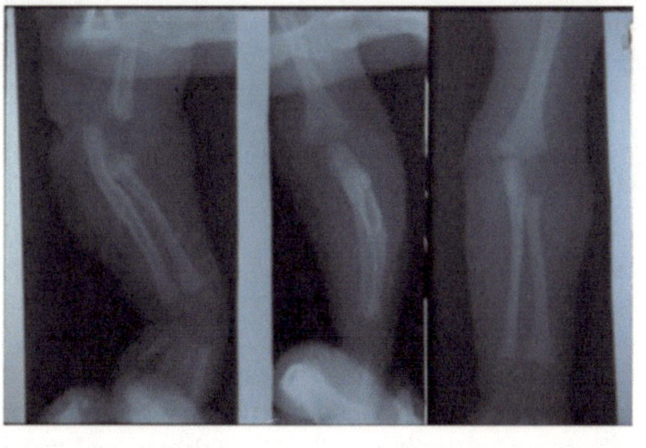

Figure 23.
Hyperostosis of the forearm (Caffey disease). Initial X-ray with periosteal reaction and plastic deformation of the radius and ulna on the right side, while the left forearm is normal. The radiological appearance at 1 year, showing widening of the forearm bones.

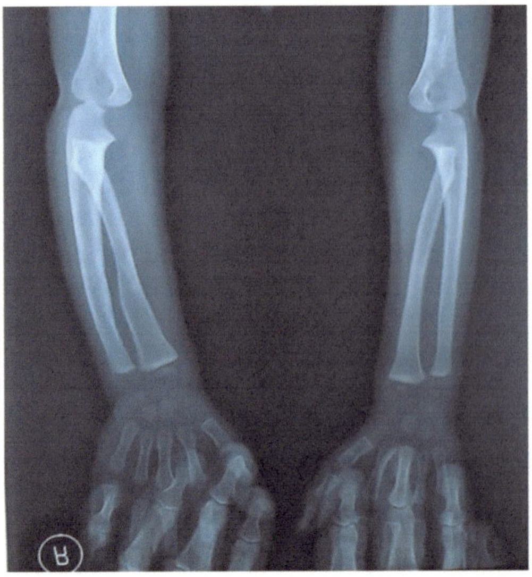

Figure 24.
Hyperostosis of the forearm (Caffey disease). Initial X-ray with periosteal reaction and plastic deformation of the radius and ulna on the right side, while the left forearm is normal. The radiological appearance at 1 year, showing widening of the forearm bones.

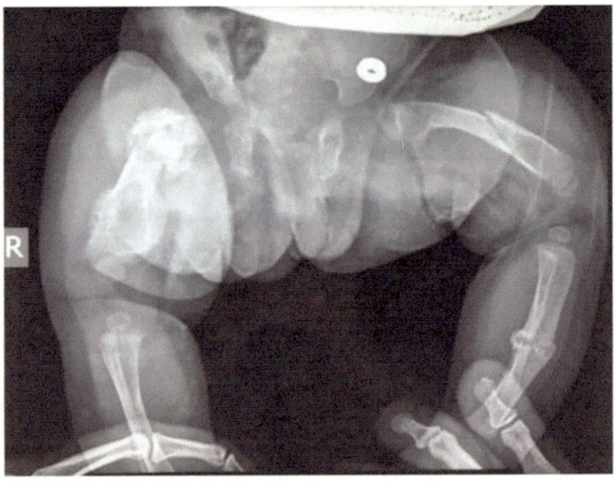

Figure 25.
Multiple fractures of femur (right with callus formation, spiral left femoral fracture and tibia left). X-rays at birth and at 3 months. At the age of 2 yrs, there are no more fractures reported. The toddler is low height.

Metaphyseal greenstick type of fracture may be found as a result of vigorous handling of the leg of the neonate. They are differentiated from cases of fibrocartilaginous bowing that are usually found during the standing period of the infant. Constriction band syndrome with tibia and fibula fracture has also been reported. Congenital pseudoarthrosis of the tibia or fibula is diagnosed rarely in the neonatal period as part of the neurofibromatosis, presenting with anteromedial bowing. Congenital posterolateral bowing of the leg is a congenital benign deformity that is not correlated with a fracture [29, 66, 71–73].

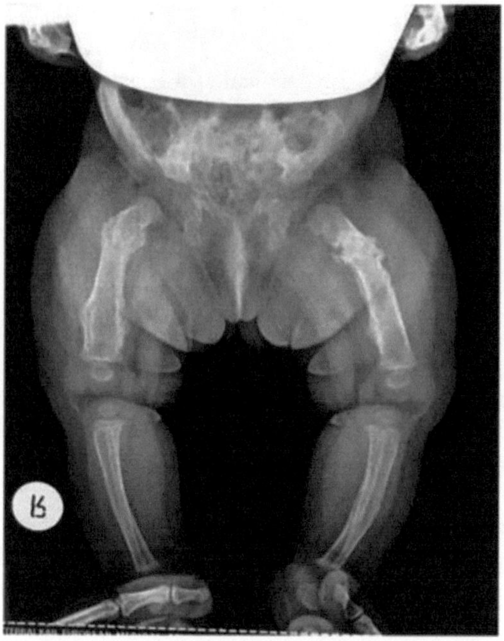

Figure 26.
Multiple fractures of femur (right with callus formation, spiral left femoral fracture and tibia left). X-rays at birth and at 3 months. At the age of 2 yrs, there are no more fractures reported. The toddler is low height.

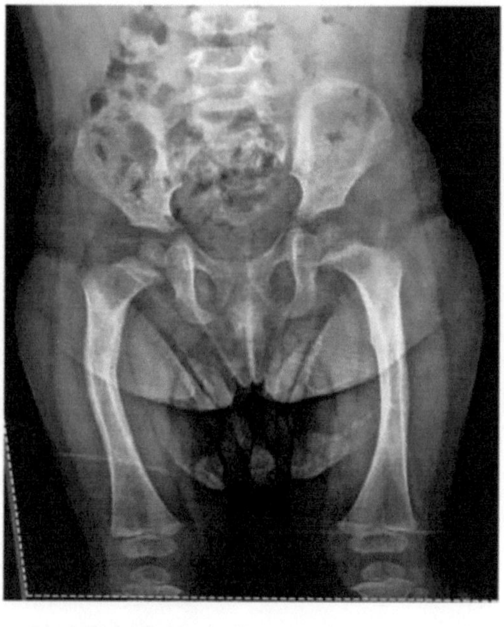

Figure 27.
Multiple fractures of femur (right with callus formation, spiral left femoral fracture and tibia left). X-rays at birth and at 3 months. At the age of 2 yrs, there are no more fractures reported. The toddler is low height.

11. Vertebral fractures

Severe spinal lesions affecting the cervical spine are extremely rare and affecting mainly the spinal cord and not the vertebrae. There are severe lesions associated with paralysis and they are usually lethal. Fractures of the vertebrae are found in neonates in severe lethal cases of OI and phosphatasia [74–77].

12. Conclusion

Neonatal fractures are reported affecting all parts of the skeleton. Their incidence is increased in cases of difficult labor with an overweight neonate. Cesarean delivery in an emergency is associated with higher incidence of long bone fractures. Neonates with an underlying disease with bone fragility sustain neonatal fractures. Fractures may also appear in uncomplicated normal labor.

Clavicle fractures are the most common and their management is appropriate handling of the neonate. Callus formation that is diagnosed later as a prominence in the clavicular area is often the main symptom. Fractures of the femur and humerus are severe complications that require appropriate treatment from a pediatric orthopedic surgeon. Diseases with bone fragility must be ruled out. Premature babies with low birth weight are at increased risk to sustain fractures. Diagnosis of epiphysiolisthesis of the distal femur and humerus is extremely difficult and appropriate reduction is essential for the management. Neonatal fractures are complications of the labor that occasionally lead to severe medicolegal problems.

Author details

Nikolaos Laliotis
Pediatric Orthopaedics, Inter Balkan Medical Center, Thessaloniki, Greece

*Address all correspondence to: nicklaliotis@gmail.com

References

[1] Groenendaal F, Hukkelhoven C. Fractures in full-term neonates. Nederlands Tijdschrift voor Geneeskunde. 2007;**151**(7):424

[2] Rehm A, Promod P, Ogilvy-Stuart A. Neonatal birth fractures: A retrospective tertiary maternity hospital review. Journal of Obstetrics and Gynaecology. 2020;**40**(4):485-490. DOI: 10.1080/01443615.2019.1631770

[3] Högberg U, Fellman V, Thiblin I, Karlsson R, Wester K. Difficult birth is the main contributor to birth-related fracture and accidents to other neonatal fractures. Acta Paediatrica. 2020;**109**(10):2040-2048. DOI: 10.1111/apa.15217

[4] Gupta R, Cabacungan ET. Neonatal birth trauma: Analysis of yearly trends, risk factors, and outcomes. The Journal of Pediatrics. 2021;**238**:174-180.e3. DOI: 10.1016/j.jpeds.2021.06.080

[5] Ariyawatkul T, Worawuthangkul K, Chotigavanichaya C, Kaewpornsawan K, Chalayon O, Eamsobhana P. Potential risk factors for birth fractures: A case-control study. International Orthopaedics. 2017;**41**(11):2361-2364. DOI: 10.1007/s00264-017-3600-5

[6] Williams BA, Makarewich CA, Montoya-Williams DC, Krakow A, Lioy J, Horn BD. Epidemiology and management of appendicular fractures occurring in neonatal intensive care patients. Acta Paediatrica. 2021;**110**(2):489-494. DOI: 10.1111/apa.15430

[7] Bhat BV, Kumar A, Oumachigui A. Bone injuries during delivery. Indian Journal of Pediatrics. 1994;**61**(4):401-405. DOI: 10.1007/BF02751901

[8] Tsai A, Grant PE, Warfield SK, Ou Y, Kleinman PK. Deep learning of birth-related infant clavicle fractures: A potential virtual consultant for fracture dating. Pediatric Radiology. 2022;**52**(11):2206-2214. DOI: 10.1007/s00247-022-05380-0

[9] Asena M, Akelma H, Ziyadanoğulları MO. The relationship between the location of neonatal clavicular fractures and predisposing factors. Journal Neonatal and Perinatal Medicine. 2020;**13**(4):507-511. DOI: 10.3233/NPM-190321

[10] Mumtaz Hashmi H, Shamim N, Kumar V, Anjum N, Ahmad K. Clavicular fractures in newborns: What happens to one of the commonly injured bones at birth? Cureus. 2021;**13**(9):e18372. DOI: 10.7759/cureus.18372

[11] Fadell M, Miller A, Trefan L, Weinman J, Stewart J, Hayes K, et al. Radiological features of healing in newborn clavicular fractures. European Radiology. 2017;**27**(5):2180-2187. DOI: 10.1007/s00330-016-4569-y

[12] Kekki M, Salonen A, Koukkula T, Laivuori H, Tihtonen K, Huttunen TT. Incidence changes in risk factors associated with the decreasing number of birth-related clavicle fractures in Finland: A nationwide retrospective birth cohort from 2004 to 2017. Birth. 2022;**00**:1-10. Jun 23. DOI: 10.1111/birt.12662

[13] Choi HA, Lee YK, Ko SY, Shin SM. Neonatal clavicle fracture in cesarean delivery: Incidence and risk factors. The Journal of Maternal-Fetal & Neonatal Medicine. 2017;**30**(14):1689-1692. DOI: 10.1080/14767058.2016.1222368

[14] Gandhi RA, DeFrancesco CJ, Shah AS. The association of clavicle

fracture with brachial plexus birth palsy. The Journal of Hand Surgery. 2019; **44**(6):467-472. DOI: 10.1016/j.jhsa.2018.11.006

[15] Laliotis NA, Chrysanthou C, Anastasopoulos N. Spontaneous union of bilateral congenital pseudoarthrosis of the clavicle, in a baby. Journal of Clinical Orthopoedic Trauma. 2020;**11**(2): 314-316. DOI: 10.1016/j.jcot.2019.04.008

[16] Fontoura-Matias J, Vilan A. Clavicle lump: Not always a fracture - A case of congenital pseudoarthrosis. Pediatrics International. 2021;**63**(12):1544-1545. DOI: 10.1111/ped.14924

[17] Pavone V, Vescio A, Montemagno M, de Cristo C, Lucenti L, Pavone P, et al. Perinatal femoral fracture: A ten-year observational case series study. Children (Basel). 2020; **7**(10):156. DOI: 10.3390/children7100156

[18] Kancherla R, Sankineani SR, Naranje S, Rijal L, Kumar R, Ansari T, et al. Birth-related femoral fracture in newborns: Risk factors and management. Journal of Children Orthopedics. 2012; **6**(3):177-180. DOI: 10.1007/s11832-012-0412-4

[19] Basha A, Amarin Z, Abu-Hassan F. Birth-associated long-bone fractures. International Journal of Gynecologic Obstetrics. 2013;**123**(2):127-130. DOI: 10.1016/j.ijgo.2013.05.013

[20] von Heideken J, Thiblin I, Högberg U. The epidemiology of infant shaft fractures of femur or humerus by incidence, birth, accidents, and other causes. BMC Musculoskeletal Disorders. 2020;**21**(1):840. DOI: 10.1186/s12891-020-03856-4

[21] Kellner KR. Neonatal fracture and cesarean section. American Journal of Diseases of Children. 1982;**136**(9):865. DOI: 10.1001/archpedi.1982.03970450107027

[22] Kanai Y, Honda Y, Honda T, Sanpei M. Delayed birth-related femur fracture after cesarean section: A case report. AJP Reports. 2018; **8**(3):e158-e160. DOI: 10.1055/s-0038-1667190

[23] Matthews JJ, Cox PJ. Gallow's traction in an incubator for treatment of neonatal femoral fracture. Annals of the Royal College of Surgeons of England. 2008;**90**(1):74-75. DOI: 10.1308/rcsann.2008.90.1.74

[24] Frik S. Management of birth-associated subtrochanteric femur fractures. Acta Orthopaedica Belgica. 2016;**82**(4):850-853

[25] D'Andrea L, Catena N. Femural shaft fracture in a newborn infant treated with axial external fixator: A case report. Journal of Pediatric Orthopedics. 2008; **28**(1):17-19. DOI: 10.1097/bpo.0b013e31815b4dea

[26] Bellur S, Jain M, Cuthbertson D, Krakow D, Shapiro JR, Steiner RD, et al. Cesarean delivery is not associated with decreased at-birth fracture rates in osteogenesis imperfecta. Genetics in Medicine. 2016;**18**(6):570-576. DOI: 10.1038/gim.2015.131

[27] Cubert R, Cheng EY, Mack S, Pepin MG, Byers PH. Osteogenesis imperfecta: Mode of delivery and neonatal outcome. Obstetrics and Gynecology. 2001;**97**(1):66-69. DOI: 10.1016/s0029-7844(00)01100-5

[28] Tournis S, Dede AD. Osteogenesis imperfecta - A clinical update. Metabolism. 2018;**80**:27-37. DOI: 10.1016/j.metabol.2017.06.001

[29] Bayram S, Mert L, Anarat FB, Chodza M, Ergin ÖN. A newborn with multiple fractures in osteogenesis imperfecta: A case report. Journal of Orthopedic Case Report. 2018;**8**(3): 71-73. DOI: 10.13107/jocr.2250-0685.1116

[30] Hackley L, Merritt L. Osteogenesis imperfecta in the neonate. Advances in Neonatal Care. 2008;**8**(1): 21-30. DOI: 10.1097/01.ANC.00003 11013.71510.41

[31] Botor M, Fus-Kujawa A, Uroczynska M, Stepien KL, Galicka A, Gawron K, et al. Osteogenesis imperfecta: Current and prospective therapies. Biomolecules. 2021;**11**(10): 1493. DOI: 10.3390/biom11101493

[32] Rao R, Cuthbertson D, Nagamani SCS, Sutton VR, Lee BH, Krischer J, et al. Pregnancy in women with osteogenesis imperfecta: Pregnancy characteristics, maternal, and neonatal outcomes. American Journal of Obstetetics and Gynecology MFM. 2021; **3**(4):100362. DOI: 10.1016/j.ajogmf. 2021.100362

[33] Sillence DO, Morley K, Ault JE. Clinical management of osteogenesis imperfecta. Connective Tissue Research. 1995;**31**(4):S15-S21. DOI: 10.3109/ 03008209509116827

[34] Deguchi M, Tsuji S, Katsura D, Kasahara K, Kimura F, Murakami T. Current overview of osteogenesis imperfecta. Medicina (Kaunas, Lithuania). 2021;**57**(5):464. DOI: 10.3390/medicina57050464

[35] Götherström C, David AL, Walther-Jallow L, Åström E, Westgren M. Mesenchymal stem cell therapy for osteogenesis imperfecta. Clinical Obstetrics and Gynecology. 2021;**64**(4): 898-903. DOI: 10.1097/GRF.00000 00000000656

[36] Laliotis N, Tsoni K, Konstantinidis P, Agakidou E, Chrysanthou C. Bilateral femoral fractures during birth, in a neonate with malformation complex with stiffness. Clinical Case Report. 2020;**8**(7):1230-1233. DOI: 10.1002/ ccr3.2877.

[37] Chinoy A, Mughal MZ, Padidela R. Metabolic bone disease of prematurity: Causes, recognition, prevention, treatment and long-term consequences. Achieves of Diseases Child Fetal Neonatal Edition. 2019;**104**(5):F560-F566. DOI: 10.1136/archdischild-2018-316330

[38] Rayannavar A, Calabria AC. Screening for metabolic bone disease of prematurity. Seminars in Fetal Neonatal Medicine 2020;**25**(1):101086. 10.1016/ j.siny.2020.101086

[39] Michaud J, Luu TM, LeBlanc JC, Healy-Profitós J, Ayoub A, Auger N. Preterm birth and the future risk of orthopedic fracture. Pediatric Research. 2020;**88**(3):466-472. DOI: 10.1038/ s41390-020-0771-3

[40] Chacham S, Pasi R, Chegondi M, Ahmad N, Mohanty SB. Metabolic bone disease in premature neonates: An unmet challenge. Journal of Clinical Research Pediatric Endocrinology. 2020; **12**(4):332-339. DOI: 10.4274/jcrpe. galenos.2019.2019.0091

[41] Schachinger F, Farr S. The effects of preterm birth on musculoskeletal health-related disorders. Journal of Clinical Medicine. 2021;**10**(21):5082. DOI: 10.3390/jcm10215082

[42] Nunes ME. In: Adam MP, Everman DB, Mirzaa GM, Pagon RA, Wallace SE, LJH B, Gripp KW,

Amemiya A, editors. Hypophosphatasia. Seattle (WA): University of Washington; 2007

[43] Laliotis N, Kapetanakis S, Gkasdaris G, Konstantinidis P, Karoutsou R, Chourmouzi D, et al. Salter-Harris type II fracture of the distal femur in a newborn: Acute anatomic imaging alterations after labor dystocia. Clinical Case Report. 2019;7(7): 1450-1451. DOI: 10.1002/ccr3.2149

[44] Franco A, Chaturvedi A. Neonatal distal femoral physeal injury secondary to mechanical trauma of birth: A case report. Clinical Imaging. 2018;**51**:65-67. DOI: 10.1016/j.clinimag.2018.02.006

[45] Eliahou R, Simanovsky N, Hiller N, Simanovsky N. Fracture-separation of the distal femoral epiphysis in a premature neonate. Journal of Ultrasound in Medicine. 2006;**25**(12): 1603-1605. DOI: 10.7863/jum.2006.25.12.1603

[46] Banagale RC, Kuhns LR. Traumatic separation of the distal femoral epiphysis in the newborn. Journal of Pediatric Orthopedics. 1983;**3**(3):396-398. DOI: 10.1097/01241398-198307000-00024

[47] Ozturk M, Yurtbay A, Keskin D, Polat AV, Selcuk MB. Subperiosteal hemorrhage due to a distal femoral physeal fracture in a neonate. North Clinical Istanbul. 2018;**6**(3):312-314. DOI: 10.14744/nci.2018.26566.article

[48] Wu X, Xia J, Li J, Sun J, Shen X. Distal femoral physeal fractures after neonatal osteomyelitis: A case report. Medicine (Baltimore). 2019;**98**(18):e15396. DOI: 10.1097/MD.0000000000015396

[49] Goyal ND, Pahwa AH, Rathod J, Jeyaraman M, Jain S, Dungarwal S. Diaphyseal fracture of the humerus during elective cesarean section - A rare case report. Journal of Orthopedic Case Report. 2021;**11**(6):10-13. DOI: 10.13107/jocr.2021.v11.i06.2236

[50] Canpolat FE, Köse A, Yurdakök M. Bilateral humerus fracture in a neonate after cesarean delivery. Archives of Gynecology and Obstetrics. 2010;**281**(5): 967-969. DOI: 10.1007/s00404-009-1256-0

[51] Kaya B, Daglar K, Kirbas A, Tüten A. Humerus diaphysis fracture in a newborn during vaginal breech delivery. Obstetrics and Gynecology. 2015;**2015**: 489108. DOI: 10.1155/2015/489108

[52] Rahul P, Grover AR, Ajoy SM. Bilateral humerus and right femur fracture in a newborn after cesarean section for breech presentation in a twin pregnancy: A very rare case report. Journal of Orthopedic Case Report. 2017; **7**(1):9-11. DOI: 10.13107/jocr.2250-0685.664

[53] Sherr-Lurie N, Bialik GM, Ganel A, Schindler A, Givon U. Fractures of the humerus in the neonatal period. The Israel Medical Association Journal. 2011; **13**(6):363-365

[54] Kumar N. Neonatal humerus shaft fracture appropriate treatment method. Medical Journal, Armed Forces India. 2005;**61**(2):210. DOI: 10.1016/S0377-1237(05)80049-8

[55] Mahapatra SK, Jangira V, Kalra M. Neonatal radial nerve palsy associated with humerus fracture: Is the fracture to be blamed? Orthopaedic Surgery. 2014; **6**(2):162-164. DOI: 10.1111/os.12106

[56] Gigante C, Kini SG, Origo C, Volpin A. Transphyseal separation of the distal humerus in newborns. Chinese Journal of Traumatology. 2017;**20**(3):183-186. DOI: 10.1016/j.cjtee.2017.04.003

[57] Malik S, Khopkar SR, Korday CS, Jadhav SS, Bhaskar AR. Transphyseal injury of distal humerus: A commonly missed diagnosis in neonates. Journal of Clinical Diagnostic Research. 2015;**9**(11): SD01-SD02. DOI: 10.7860/JCDR/2015/11619.6715

[58] Patil MN, Palled E. Epihyseal separation of lower end humerus in a neonate-diagnostic and management difficulty. Journal of Orthopedic Case Report. 2015;**5**(4):7-9. DOI: 10.13107/jocr.2250-0685.332

[59] Kamaci S, Danisman M, Marangoz S. Neonatal physeal separation of distal humerus during cesarean section. American Journal of Orthopedic. 2014; **43**(11):E279-W281

[60] Supakul N, Hicks RA, Caltoum CB, Karmazyn B. Distal humeral epiphyseal separation in young children: An often-missed fracture-radiographic signs and ultrasound confirmatory diagnosis. AJR. American Journal of Roentgenology. 2015;**204**(2):W192-W198. DOI: 10.2214/AJR.14.12788

[61] Jacobsen S, Hansson G, Nathorst-Westfelt J. Traumatic separation of the distal epiphysis of the humerus sustained at birth. Journal of Bone and Joint Surgery. British Volume (London). 2009;**91**(6):797-802. DOI: 10.1302/0301-620X.91B6.22140

[62] Tharakan SJ, Lee RJ, White AM, Lawrence JT. Distal humeral epiphyseal separation in a newborn. Orthopedics. 2016;**39**(4):e764-e767. DOI: 10.3928/01477447-20160503-01

[63] Sabat D, Maini L, Gautam VK. Neonatal separation of distal humeral epiphysis during Caesarean section: A case report. Journal of Orthopaedic Surgery (Hong Kong). 2011;**19**(3): 376-378. DOI: 10.1177/230949901101900325

[64] Ratti C, Guindani N, Riva G, Callegari L, Grassi FA, Murena L. Transphyseal elbow fracture in newborn: Review of literature. Musculoskeletal Surgery. 2015;**99**(Suppl. 1):S99-S105. DOI: 10.1007/s12306-015-0366-z

[65] Kay M, Simpkins C, Shipman P, Whitewood C. Diagnosing neonatal transphyseal fractures of the distal humerus. Journal of Medical Imaging and Radiation Oncology. 2017; **61**(4):494-499. DOI: 10.1111/1754-9485.12607

[66] Laliotis N. Bone lesions in children with neurofibromatosis. In: Book Neurofibromatosis. London, UK: Intechopen; 2021. DOI: 10.5772/intechopen.97802

[67] Koo WW, Sherman R, Succop P, Oestreich AE, Tsang RC, Krug-Wispe SK, et al. Sequential bone mineral content in small preterm infants with and without fractures and rickets. Journal of Bone and Mineral Research. 1988;**3**(2):193-197. DOI: 10.1002/jbmr.5650030211

[68] Angelis S, Vynichakis G, Trellopoulos A, Mirtsios H, Michelarakis JN. Trangling congenital constriction ring band of the forearm with fracture: A rare case report. Cureus. 2019;**11**(3): e4189. DOI: 10.7759/cureus.4189

[69] Nistala H, Mäkitie O, Jüppner H. Caffey disease: New perspectives on old questions. Bone. 2014;**60**:264-251. DOI: 10.1016/j.bone.2013.12.030

[70] Elfatairy KK, Ehrlich L, Porrino J, Wang A. Congenital pseudarthrosis of the forearm as a single manifestation of neurofibromatosis type 1 at birth: A case report. Clinical Imaging. 2021;**78**: 214-216. DOI: 10.1016/j.clinimag.2021.04.032

[71] Lee GS, Methratta ST, Frasier LD. Classic metaphyseal lesion of distal tibia following footling breech delivery. Pediatric Radiology. 2019;**49**(13): 1840-1842. DOI: 10.1007/s00247-019-04490-6

[72] Lysack JT, Soboleski D. Classic metaphyseal lesion following external cephalic version and cesarean section. Pediatric Radiology. 2003;**33**(6):422-424. DOI: 10.1007/s00247-003-0914-9

[73] Kaplan M, Dollberg M, Wajntraub G, Itzchaki M. Fractured long bones in a term infant delivered by cesarian section. Pediatric Radiology. 1987;**17**(3):256-257. DOI: 10.1007/BF02388179

[74] Vialle R, Piétin-Vialle C, Ilharreborde B, Dauger S, Vinchon M, Glorion C. Spinal cord injuries at birth: A multicenter review of nine cases. Maternal Fetal and Neonatal Medicine. 2007;**20**(6):435-440. DOI: 10.1080/14767050701288325

[75] Caird MS, Reddy S, Ganley TJ, Drummond DS. Cervical spine fracture-dislocation birth injury: Prevention, recognition, and implications for the orthopaedic surgeon. Journal of Pediatric Orthopedics. 2005;**25**(4):484-486. DOI: 10.1097/01.bpo.0000158006.61294.ff

[76] Menticoglou SM, Perlman M, Manning FA. High cervical spinal cord injury in neonates delivered with forceps: Report of 15 cases. Obstetrics and Gynecology. 1995;**86**(4 Pt 1): 589-594. DOI: 10.1016/0029-7844(95)00213-b

[77] Lee CC, Chou IJ, Chang YJ, Chiang MC. Unusual presentations of birth related cervical spinal cord injury. Frontiers in Pediatrics. 2020;**8**:514. DOI: 10.3389/fped.2020.00514

Chapter 3

Intramedullary Fixation of Midshaft Clavicle Fractures

Martin D. Richardson and Louise M. Richardson

Abstract

Midshaft clavicle fractures are a common orthopaedic upper limb injury in young athletes and in trauma. While non-operative care has traditionally been the preferred therapeutic approach, surgical intervention is becoming more popular, to improve patient outcomes and speed the return to function. Intramedullary screw fixation has developed as a successful surgical treatment for midshaft clavicle fractures, in recent years, giving greater stability and encouraging early mobilisation. This chapter provides an overview of the efficacy, complications, and clinical outcomes of intramedullary screw treatment for midshaft clavicle fractures. According to current research, intra-medullary screw fixation has various advantages over standard non-operative therapy, including increased fracture stability, lower non-union rates, and improved functional outcomes. Complications from this procedure, such as implant migration or discomfort, are often minor and controllable. However, careful patient selection, preoperative preparation, and surgical expertise are required to achieve the best results.

Keywords: midshaft clavicle fracture, intramedullary fixation, common upper limb injury, significantly displaced, shortened

1. Introduction

Clavicle fractures are very common, accounting for 2.6–4% of all fractures [1, 2]. The majority of these, greater than 80%, occur in the midshaft [3]. They are commonly associated with athletic activities such as contact sports (such as football), cycling, and snow sports, and occur typically in a younger male patient group [2]. Undisplaced fractures are usually treated non-operatively, but indications for operative treatment have led to a general consensus that displacement and/or shortening of greater than 20 mm leads to a higher mal-union and non-union rate and is a stronger indication for operative treatment. Zlowodzki et al. [4] reported a 15.1% non-union rate for non-operatively treated displaced clavicle fractures. They identified factors associated with nonunion including displacement, comminution, female sex, and increased age. Postacchini et al. [2] noted 48% of fractures in their study were displaced and 19% were comminuted. This chapter outlines a surgical approach for intramedullary fixation of midshaft clavicle fractures using a cannulated intramedullary screw. A recent systematic review supported a lower incidence of nonunion and symptomatic malunion in patients who underwent operative fixation of displaced midshaft clavicular fractures compared to conservative management [5].

Furthermore, there is mounting evidence that intramedullary fixation achieves similar or superior functional outcomes to plate fixation, but with lower complication rates [6]. The decision to proceed with operative management will be patient specific and will be affected by factors such as: deformity, disability, patient choice, the local health care system, implant cost and availability, and the overall relative cost/benefit of the procedure. For instance, operative fixation for a tradesperson, dependent on upper limb use, may allow substantially more rapid return to work and reduced off-work costs.

2. Variety of intramedullary devices

Numerous implants have been used to fix midshaft clavicular fractures by an intra-medullary technique.

2.1 Kirschner wires

There have been accounts of successful K-wire stabilisation of clavicle fractures since the early 1940s [7]. However, Lyons and Rockwood [8] cautioned that Implants around the shoulder girdle that have the potential to migrate and end up in cerebral or intrathoracic structures can have severe adverse effects.

2.2 Titanium elastic nails (TENs)

TENS were originally developed to manage paediatric long bone fractures without causing damage to the epiphyses and have been used to manage midshaft clavicular fractures, with one benefit being a MIPO approach that minimises surgical scars [9]. The inability to manage the implant's length and rotation are potential drawbacks of this method. This restricts their application to more simple configurations, such as transverse or short oblique fractures with minimal comminution [10]. Significant radiation from the C-arm is required to handle the implant with an image intensifier (fluoroscopy), exposing both patient and operators to increased radiation exposure. Additionally, Jubel et al. [11] reported a 15 mm loss of length in the post-operative period following comminuted fracture fixation. Frigg et al. [12] reported a complication rate of 70% and 36% revision rate, using this approach. In this group 44% of the fractures were comminuted. Randomised controlled trials comparing TENs to plate fixation [13, 14] showed high union rates (96–100%) but also significant complication rates (over 60%).

2.3 Hagie pins

The San Antonio -based Rockwood team described the use of a Modified Rockwood-Hagie pin for treating midshaft clavicular non-unions [15]. This device has been used successfully by a number of groups, with union rates ranging from 91.4 to 100% [16–20]. Mudd et al. [21] reported less favourable results in a small study, with an 83.3% (15/18) union rate. All authors reported that irritation from the prominent lateral end of the implant necessitated removal.

In our experience with this device, the inability to have the length less than 120 mm resulted in prominence of the nuts on the lateral side and often protrusion of the medial end of the screw anteriorly, causing subcuticular irritation, requiring implant removal. We have since chosen devices with more length options that can be made completely intra-osseous, avoiding a second operation to remove the implant. This is also a common problem when plates are used. As the clavicle lies in a subcutaneous plane with little soft tissue and muscular coverage, extra-osseous implants will frequently cause irritation and necessitate a second procedure for removal.

2.4 Knowles pins

Knowles pins are solid threaded nails used to repair midshaft clavicular fractures [22]. Unfortunately, due to their length, one or both ends of the pin frequently protrude from the bone, causing irritation requiring removal after fracture healing.

2.5 Echidna pins

Echidna pins (**Figure 1**) were developed to aid rotational and length stability [23, 24]. The retractable spikes on this intramedullary device can be deployed once in position to achieve fixation in the proximal and distal fragments. While experimental studies have demonstrated good biomechanical performance, this device has not been clinically trialled.

2.6 Solid intra-medullary screws

Khalil [25] described a medial to lateral approach that made use of a solid 6.5 mm screw, but the prominent medial head caused significant discomfort and additional surgery was needed for implant removal. Abo El Nor [26] used a similar device with

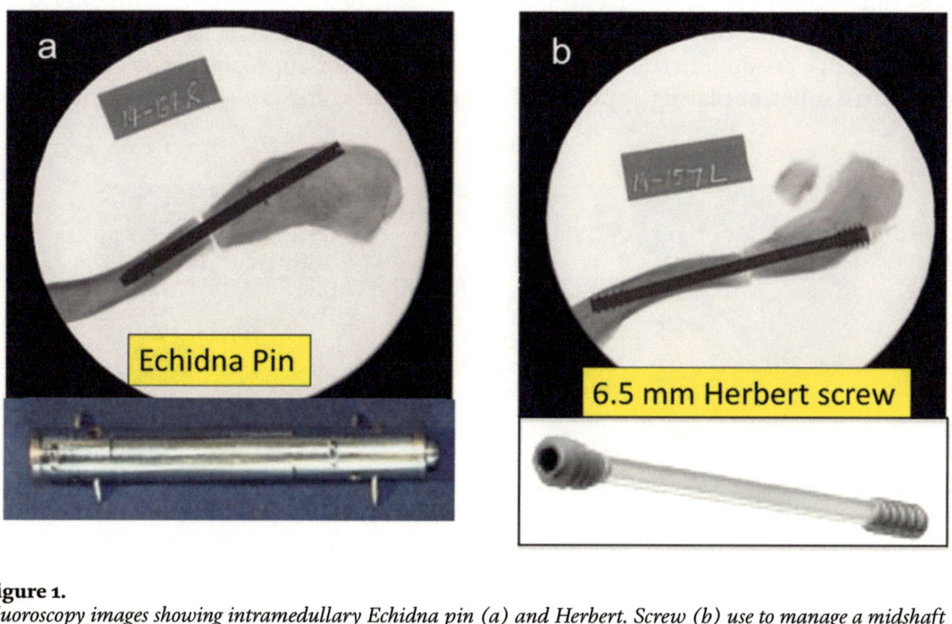

Figure 1.
Fluoroscopy images showing intramedullary Echidna pin (a) and Herbert. Screw (b) use to manage a midshaft clavicular fracture.

a lateral to medial insertion after retrograde drilling of the lateral fragment and achieved a 100% union rate while avoiding the medial head prominence.

2.7 Cannulated intra-medullary screws

Our intra-medullary fixation preference is now a cannulated intra-medullary screw (**Figure 1**) with differential threads at either end. Originally, we used 4.5 mm diameter Herbert screws for females and adolescent males and the 6.5 mm Herbert screws for most adult males. Unfortunately, these have been discontinued recently. We successfully have variants on this theme with different diameters and lengths. Typically, 70–100 mm lengths have been suitable. The advantage of this design is that temporary reduction can be made over a guide wire before definitive placement of the cannulated screw. The screw can be made completely intra-osseous reducing the likelihood of hardware irritation and the need for subsequent removal. The differential threads at either end of the screw provide length and rotational control (**Figure 2**).

3. Risks

Numerous sensory supraclavicular nerves run over the clavicle, supplying skin over the anterior chest down to the level of the nipple. The area of numbness created by the surgical approach to the clavicle is directly related to the size of the incision. Plating techniques typically require larger incisions than intramedullary approaches, resulting in a higher risk of numbness or dysthaesia.

It has been demonstrated that both the subclavian artery and vein lie very close to the inferior surface of the clavicle bone (12.2 mm and 8.3 mm, respectively) [27, 28] and are at risk of damage if a drill bit is plunged or an excessively long screw is used when plating midshaft clavicle fractures. The brachial plexus is also intimately related to the midshaft of the clavicle (within 8.3 mm). Bain et al. [29] have documented a pseudo aneurysm of the axillary artery after plating of a midshaft clavicular fracture. These findings resulted in the conclusion that an anterior approach is potentially safer than a superior plating approach. The apex of the lung is also just deep to

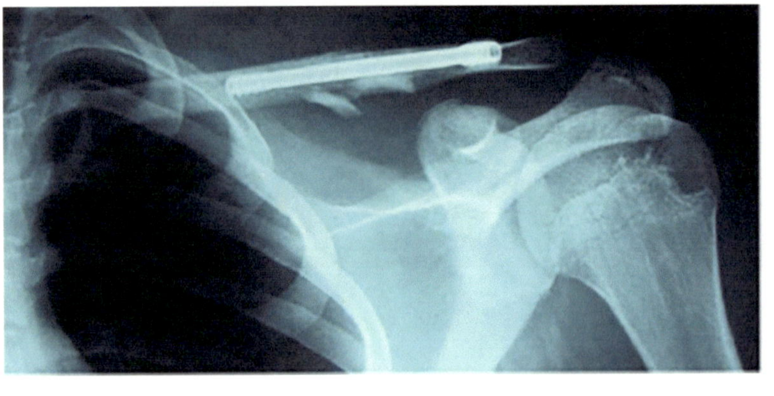

Figure 2.
Well reduced clavicle fracture with intra medullary cannulated screw with differential threaded Herbert styled screw threads to aid with fracture stabilization, compression and rotational control.

the neurovascular structures and may be at risk, with resultant pneumothorax, if damaged.

The preparation of a midshaft clavicle fracture for fixation with an intramedullary screw is done entirely within the plane of the clavicle, protecting the nearby neurovascular structures.

4. Operative technique

We have developed an operative technique which exposes the fracture directly, allowing mobilisation of the fractured ends of the midshaft clavicle and preparation of the intramedullary canal of the main shaft elements, which are essentially straight. The lateral end of the clavicle curves anteriorly to become the acromio-clavicular joint, thus lateral reaming deliberately perforates the posterior cortex behind the acromio-clavicular joint. A straight guide pin can then be directed posteriorly to allow a percutaneous incision to be made through which the pin can be pushed. The fracture can then be reduced over the pin and advanced medially into the medial fragment. The intramedullary device can be further advanced to achieve reduction and fixation of the fracture akin to similar fixations in other long bones fixed with intramedullary devices, like a midshaft tibia or femoral fracture.

If the fracture is comminuted as in the Xray in **Figure 3**, the butterfly fragments can be carefully pushed to the side maintaining their periosteal soft tissue attachments and (thus their vascularity) and sutured back into place around the reduced fracture. Bone graft can be harvested from the drill bits used to open the medullary canal, which can then be used to primarily bone graft the fracture site, promoting earlier fracture healing. The wound can then be closed in layers, first with muscular sutures and then with dermal and subcuticular dissolvable sutures to re-cover the clavicle.

Elements of the operative technique are illustrated in **Figures 4–11**, and **Figure 12** provides a stepwise diagrammatic representation of the procedure.

A more detailed demonstration video of the procedure can be accessed at Vumedi.com [30].

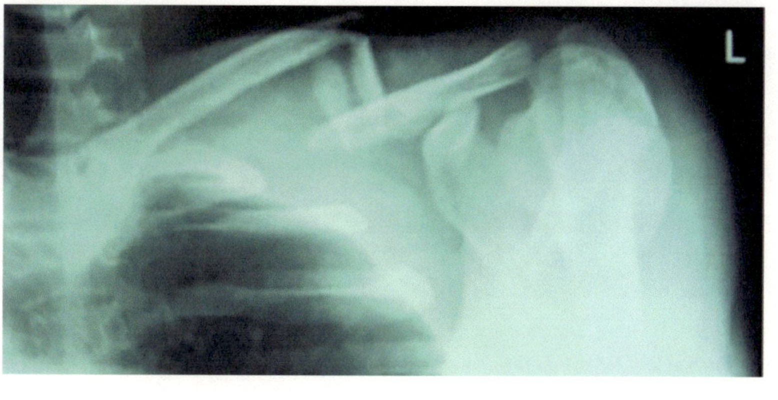

Figure 3.
Plain radiograph of a comminuted midshaft clavicular fracture, shortened and displaced more than 20mm.

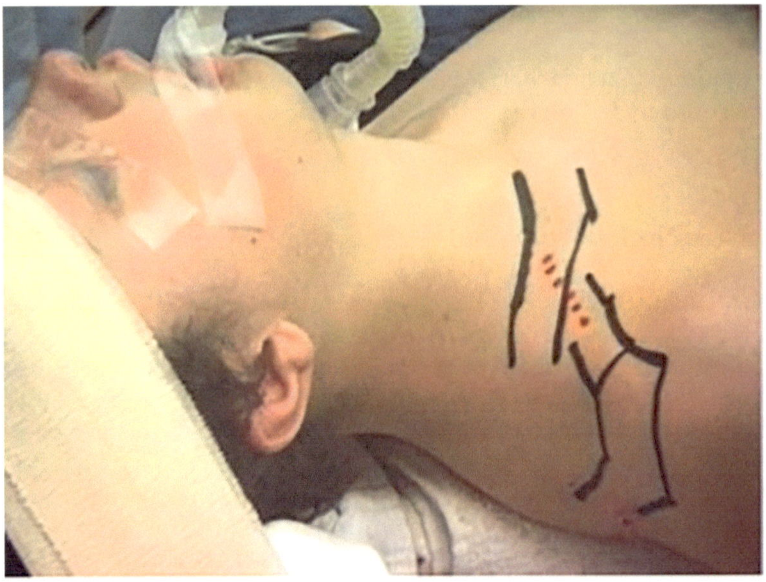

Figure 4.
Positioning of patient supine with their head on a donut ring, at the edge of the bed and secured to the table with head strapping. A rolled towel or litre bag of saline placed under scapula aids fracture reduction and arm is positioned on arm board.

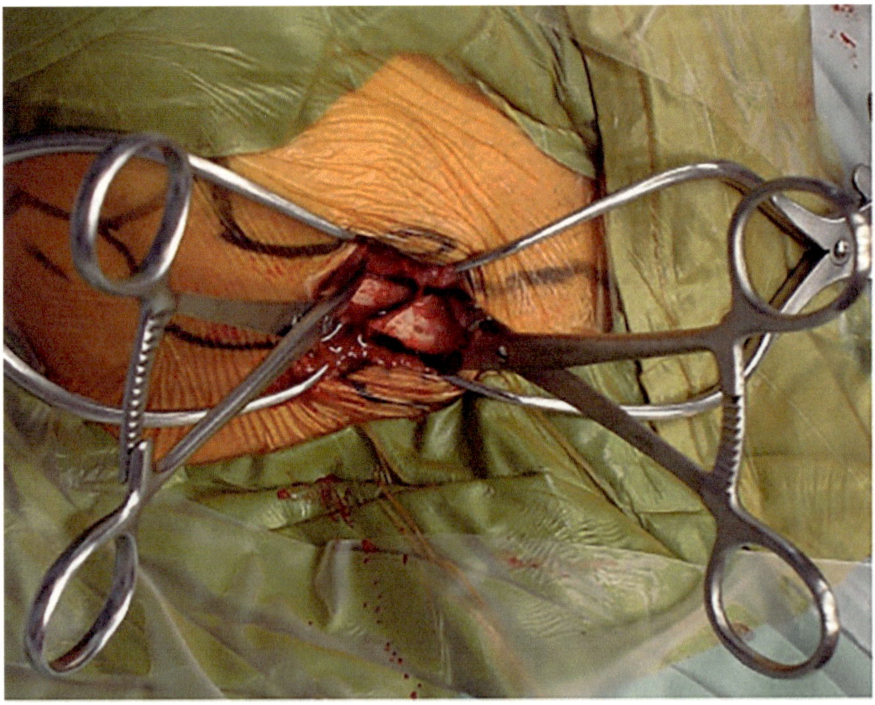

Figure 5.
Manipulation of medial and lateral shaft fragments with small fragment bone clamps to allow preparation and ultimate bony reduction.

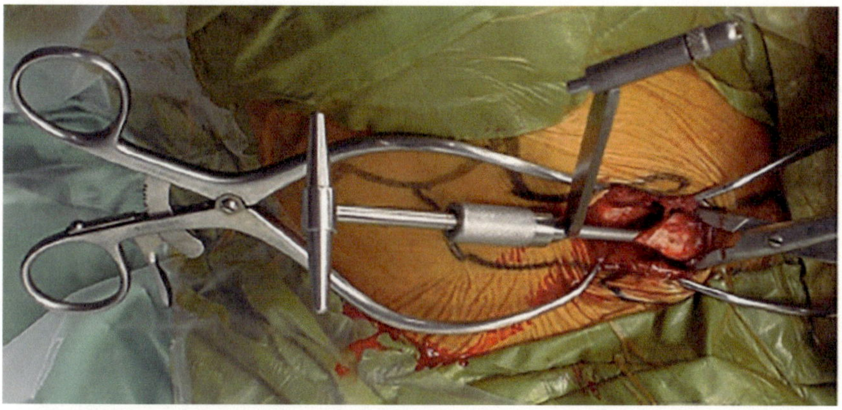

Figure 6.
Preparation of intramedullary canal with handheld drill bits.

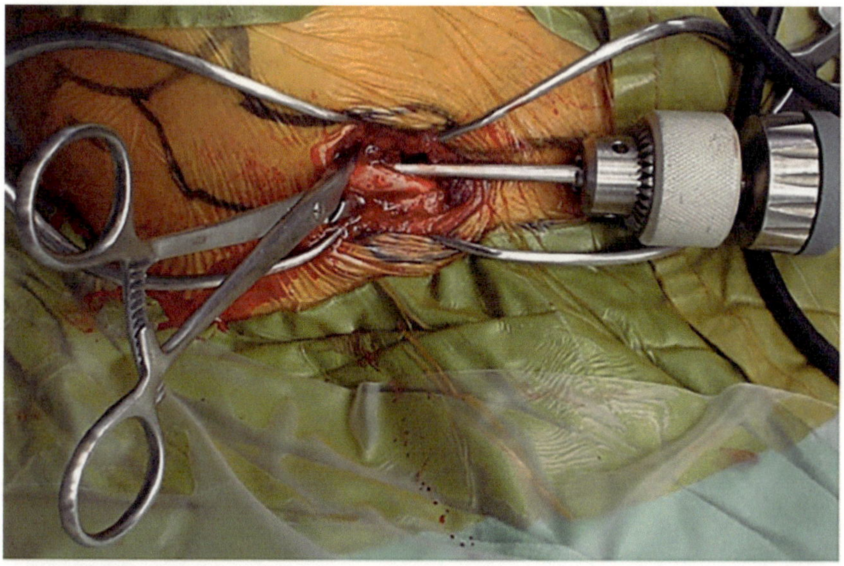

Figure 7.
Preparation of lateral fragment, initially by hand, and ultimately perforation of postero-lateral cortex with power.

5. Clinical results

Xie et al. [31] performed a systematic review of eight overlapping meta-analyses comparing the results of plate versus intra-medullary fixation of displaced midshaft clavicular fractures. While the functional or non-union outcomes did not differ between the two treatment groups, they did document a higher reintervention and refracture rate after implant removal of plate implants.

We reported on 114 of our own cases, with a 2.6% non-union rate [32]. The reoperation rate was also low (1.7%).

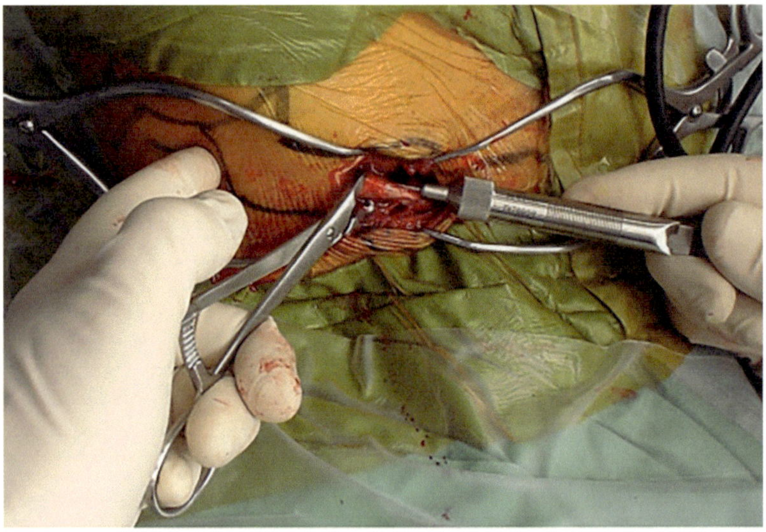

Figure 8.
Measurement of length of intramedullary fragments both medial and lateral to determine length of intramedullary device.

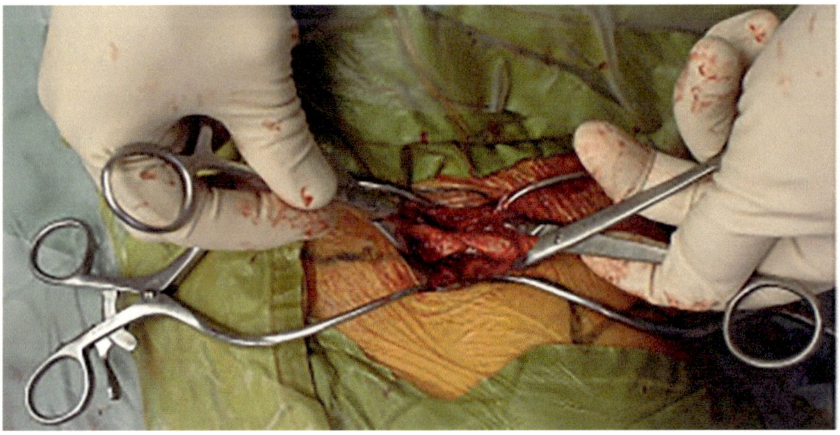

Figure 9.
Final reduction of fracture over intramedullary pin, the intramedullary device can then be inserted from the lateral percutaneous incision medially across the reduced fracture.

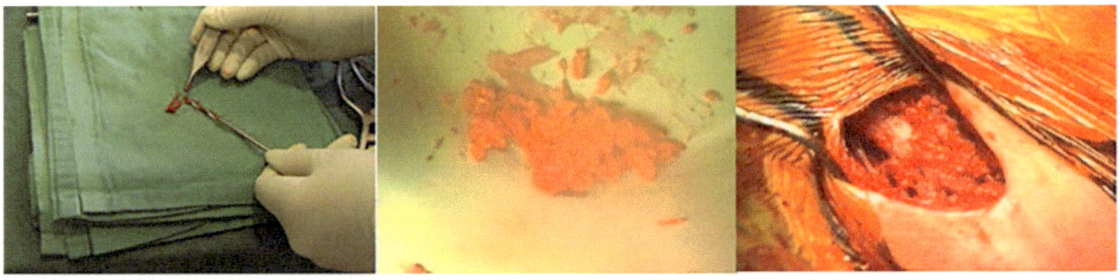

Figure 10.
Care taken to harvest reamings, from the intramedullary drills, yields abundant bone graft to be placed as primary bone graft to promote fracture healing.

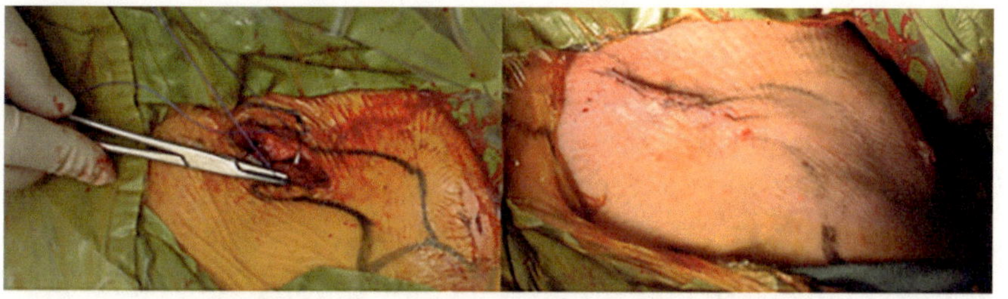

Figure 11.
Suturing of periosteal soft tissue attachments of butterfly fragments back into place around reduced fracture.

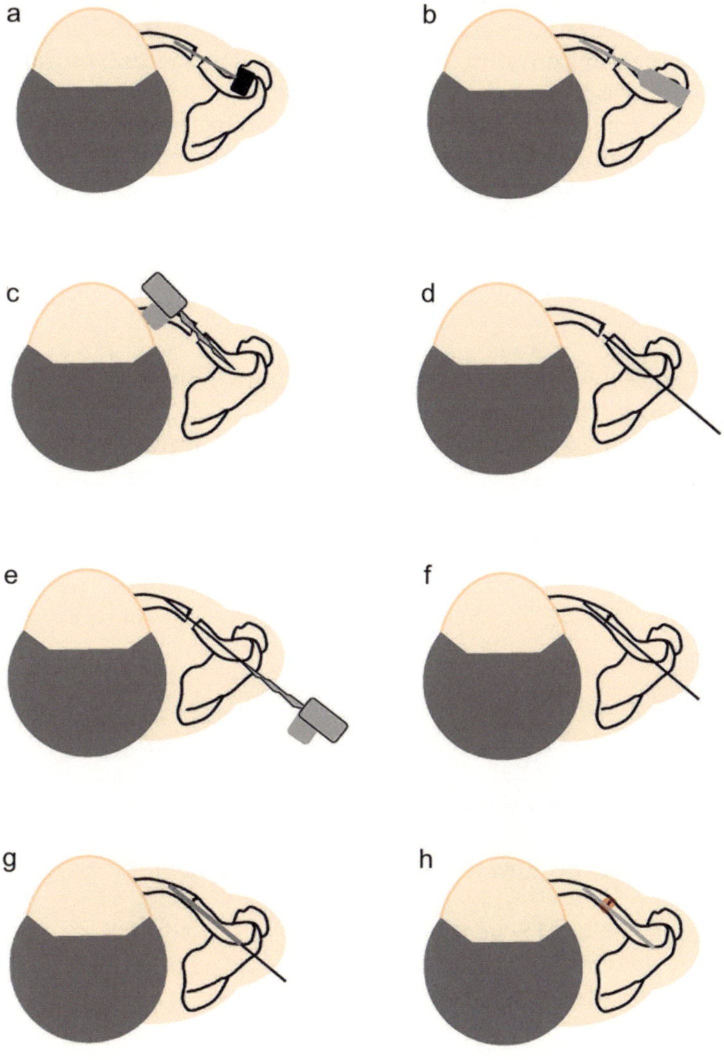

Figure 12.
Diagrammatic representation of the operative procedure. (a) Hand-drilling the intramedullary canal of the medial fragment. (b) Tapping the intramedullary canal of the medial fragment. (c) The intramedullary canal of the lateral fragment was power drilled. (d) The guide wire is introduced in retrogradely. (e) The posterolateral cortex is drilled out using a step drill. (f) Reinsertion of the guide wire and fracture reduction. (g) Placement of a cannulated Herbert screw at the fracture site. (h) Implantation of harvested bone graft around the fracture site.

6. Biomechanics

Smith et al. [33] demonstrated superior strength of clavicles fixed with an intramedullary device after removal of hardware compared to plates, raising the concern of refracture for plate fixation.

7. Treatment of delayed, mal-unions and non-unions

Treatment of midshaft clavicular fractures is easier if performed within 28 days of the fracture as much of the dissection of the fracture ends has been done by the trauma. Union rates are higher in the acute group, while complications are lower, implying that the decision to operate should ideally be made in the first month [34]. When treating a mal- or non-united mid shaft clavicular fracture, caution is required because the anatomy is likely to be distorted and adhesions may increase the risk of damage to neuro-vascular structures when osteotomizing a mal union or mobilising and debriding a non-union. Our technique of using intramedullary reamings aids the healing of these cases. A small curette is an excellent tool to locate and develop the medullary canal safely for implant insertion.

8. Conclusion

Midshaft clavicle fractures are common upper limb injuries that generally affect younger active males. The natural history of conservatively treated displaced fractures is characterised by a high mal- and non-union rate. Intra-medullary fixation of midshaft clavicle fractures provides a safe consistent method of managing these fractures, allowing early return to function in both the sporting arena and workplace.

Author details

Martin D. Richardson[1*] and Louise M. Richardson[2]

1 University of Melbourne, Epworth Hospital Clinical School, Australia

2 Epworth Hospital Clinical School, Australia

*Address all correspondence to: orthovic@gmail.com

References

[1] Nordqvist A, Petersson C. The incidence of fractures of the clavicle. Clinical Orthopaedics and Related Research. 1994;**300**:127-132

[2] Postacchini F, Gumina S, De Santis P, Albo F. Epidemiology of clavicle fractures. Journal of Shoulder and Elbow Surgery. 2002;**11**(5):452-456. DOI: 10.1067/mse.2002.126613

[3] McKee M. Clavicle fractures. In: Bucholz R, Court-Brown C, Heckman J, editors. Fractures in Adults. Lippincott: Williams & Wilkins; 2010. pp. 1106-1141

[4] Zlowodzki M, Zelle B, Cole P, Jeray K, McKee M. Treatment of acute midshaft clavicle fractures systematic review of 2144 Fractures_On behalf of the evidence-based orthopaedic trauma working group. Journal of Ortho Trauma. 2005;**19**(7):504-507

[5] Amer K, Smith B, Thomson JE, Congiusta D, Reilly MC, Sirkin MS, et al. Operative versus nonoperative outcomes of middle-third clavicle fractures: A systematic review and Meta-analysis. Journal of Orthopaedic Trauma. 2020;**34**(1):e6-e13. DOI: 10.1097/BOT.0000000000001602

[6] Hoogervorst P, van Dam T, Verdonschot N, Hannink G. Functional outcomes and complications of intramedullary fixation devices for midshaft clavicle fractures: A systematic review and meta-analysis. BMC Musculoskeletal Disorders. 2020;**21**(1):395. DOI: 10.1186/s12891-020-03256-8

[7] Murray G. A method of fixation for fracture of the clavicle. JBJS A. 1940;**22**(3):616-620

[8] Lyons F, Rockwood C. Current concepts review: Migration of pins used in operations on the shoulder. JBJS A. 1990;**72A**(8):1262-1267

[9] Fuglesang HFS, Oksum MA, Wikeroy AKB. Mini-invasive intramedullary fixation of displaced midshaft clavicle fractures with an elastic titanium nail. JBJS Essential Surgery Technology. 2018;**8**(2):e16. DOI: 10.2106/JBJS.ST.18.00001

[10] Chung HJ, Hong KJ, Kim DS. Biomechanical properties of titanium elastic nail applied to a cadaveric clavicle model. Orthopaedics & Traumatology, Surgery & Research. 2015;**101**(7):823-826. DOI: 10.1016/j.otsr.2015.06.023

[11] Jubel A, Andermahr J, Schiffer G, Tsironis K, Rehm K. Elastic stable intramedullary nailing of midclavicular fractures with a titanium nail. CORR. 2003;**408**:279-285. DOI: 10.1097/01.blo.0000048131.30533.81

[12] Frigg A, Rillmann P, Perren T, Gerber M, Ryf C. Intramedullary nailing of clavicular midshaft fractures with the titanium elastic nail: Problems and complications. The American Journal of Sports Medicine. 2009;**37**(2):352-359

[13] Andrade-Silva F, Kojima K, Joeris A, Santos SJ, Mattar R. Single, superiorly placed reconstruction plate compared with flexible intramedullary nailing for midshaft clavicular fractures: A prospective, randomized controlled trial. The Journal of Bone and Joint Surgery. American Volume. 2015;**97**(8):620-626

[14] van der Meijden O, Houwert R, Hulsmans M. Operative treatment of dislocated midshaft clavicular fractures: Plate or intramedullary nail fixation? A

randomized controlled trial. The Journal of Bone and Joint Surgery. American Volume. 2015;**97A**(8):613-619

[15] Boehme D, Curtis R, DeHaan J, Kay S, Young D, Rockwwod C. Non-union of fractures of the mid-shaft of the clavicle. Treatment with a modified Hagie intramedullary pin and autogenous bone-grafting. JBJS A. 1991;**73 A**(8):1219-1226

[16] Ferran N, Hodgson P, Vannet N, Williams R, Evans R. Locked intramedullary fixation vs plating for displaced and shortened mid-shaft clavicle fractures: A randomized clinical trial. Journal of Shoulder and Elbow Surgery. 2010;**19**(6):783-789

[17] Kleweno C, Jawa A, Wells J. Midshaft clavicular fractures: Comparison of intramedullary pin and plate fixation. Journal of Shoulder and Elbow Surgery. 2011;**20**(7):1114-1117

[18] Millett P, Hurst J, Horan M, Hawkins R. Complications of clavicle fractures treated with intramedullary fixation. Journal of Shoulder and Elbow Surgery. 2011;**20**(1):86-91

[19] Payne D, Wray W, Ruch D, Zura R, Moorman C. Outcome of intramedullary fixation of clavicular fractures. The American Journal of Orthopedics. 2011;**40**(6):E99-E104

[20] Strauss E, Egol K, France M, Koval K, Zuckerman J. Complications of intramedullary Hagie pin fixation for acute midshaft clavicle fractures. Journal of Shoulder and Elbow Surgery. 2007;**16**(3):280-284

[21] Mudd C, Quigley K, Gross L. Excessive complications of open intramedullary nailing of midshaft clavicle fractures with the Rockwood clavicle pin. Clinical Orthopaedics and Related Research. 2011;**469**(12):3364-3370

[22] Jou IM, Chiang EP, Lin CJ, Lin CL, Wang PH, Su WR. Treatment of unstable distal clavicle fractures with Knowles pin. Journal of Shoulder and Elbow Surgery. 2011;**20**(3):414-419. DOI: 10.1016/j.jse.2010.08.009

[23] Ackland D, Griggs I, Hislop P, Wu W, Patel M, Richardson M. An intramedullary Echidna pin for fixation of comminuted clavicle fractures: A biomechanical study. Journal of Orthopaedic Surgery and Research. 2017;**12**(1):122. DOI: 10.1186/s13018-017-0623-y

[24] Sidhu N, Huntington LS, Richardson M, Ackland DC. Biomechanical performance of an intramedullary Echidna pin for fixation of comminuted mid-shaft clavicle fractures. ANZ Journal of Surgery. 2019;**89**(10):1308-1313. DOI: 10.1111/ans.15392

[25] Khalil A. Intramedullary screw fixation for midshaft fractures of the clavicle. International Orthopaedics. 2009;**33**(5):1421-1424

[26] Abo El Nor T. Displaced mid-shaft clavicular fractures: Surgical treatment with intramedullary screw fixation. Archives of Orthopaedic and Trauma Surgery. 2013;**133**(10):1395-1399

[27] Galley IJ, Watts AC, Bain GI. The anatomic relationship of the axillary artery and vein to the clavicle: A cadaveric study. Journal of Shoulder and Elbow Surgery. 2009;**18**(5):e21-e25. DOI: 10.1016/j.jse.2009.01.021

[28] Hussey M, Chen Y, Fajardo R, Dutta A. Analysis of neurovascular safety between superior and anterior plating techniques of clavicle fractures. Journal of Ortho Trauma. 2013;**27**(11):627-632

[29] Bain G, Galley I, Keogh A, Durrant A. Axillary artery pseudoaneurysm after plate osteosynthesis for a clavicle nonunion: A case report and literature review. International Journal of Shoulder Surgery. 2010;**4**(3):79

[30] Richardson M. Fixation of midshaft clavicle fracture with an intra-medullary Herbert screw. VuMedi. 2019. Available from: https://www.vumedi.com/video/fixation-of-midshaft-clavicle-fracture-with-an-intra-medullary-herbert-screw/

[31] Xie L, Zhao Z, Zhang S, Hu Y. Intramedullary fixation versus plate fixation for displaced mid-shaft clavicle fractures: A systematic review of overlapping meta-analyses. Medicine (Baltimore). 2018;**97**(4):e9752. DOI: 10.1097/MD.0000000000009752

[32] Richardson M, Asadollahi S, Richardson L. Management of acute displaced clavicular fractures using Herbert cannulated screw: Technique and results in 114 patients. International Journal of Shoulder Surgery. 2013;**16**(7):1-7

[33] Smith SD, Wijdicks CA, Jansson KS, Boykin RE, Martetschlaeger F, de Meijer PP, et al. Stability of mid-shaft clavicle fractures after plate fixation versus intramedullary repair and after hardware removal. Knee Surgery, Sports Traumatology, Arthroscopy. 2014;**22**(2):448-455. DOI: 10.1007/s00167-013-2411-5

[34] Richardson M, Richardson L, Asadollahi S. Delayed surgical treatment of displaced midshaft clavicle fracture using Herbert cannulated screw with intramedullary bone graft. European Journal of Orthopaedic Surgery and Traumatology. 2012;**22**(8):647-653. DOI: 10.1007/s00590-011-0877-8

Chapter 4

Management of Distal Femoral Fractures

Luis Bahamonde and Alvaro Zamorano

Abstract

Operative treatment of distal femoral fractures has evolved significantly in tems of strategy and implants available for fracture fixation. Major advances include improvements in fixation devices, as well as the understanding of the pathomechanics of fixation failures. As the complexity of the fracture increases, and in conjunction with considerations of the general status and functionality of the patient, judicious planning, surgical approach and choice of implants can be undertaken, in order to obtain optimal functional restoration. This goes along tightly with the capability of a given construct to withstand deforming forces, while early mobilization and weight bearing take splace, and ultimately bone healing occurs. Minimizing the risk of complications, such as hardware failure and nonunion, depend closely on proper planning and execution. Factors inherent to the patient and the fracture itself are beyond the surgeon's control. But taking these in mind, allows the surgeon to select properly the timing, surgical approach and choice of implant—or combination of implants—, best suited for a given patient.

Keywords: distal femoral fractures, mechanical failure, nail, plate fixation, surgical technique

1. Introduction

Fractures of the distal part of the femur, whether extra articular or intra articular, have a bimodal distribution. At younger ages, high-energy trauma is the main cause, whereas in the elderly, low energy trauma results in a fracture due to osteopenia [1, 2]. In any case, the fracture pattern varies in terms of comminution, site of the fracture (articular and/or extraarticular), quality of bone and general condition of the patient. The high loads and bending forces affecting this anatomical area contribute to the complexity of the problem on a given patient. Hardware failure and nonunion are major concerns, and occur irrespective of the fixation method in nearly one of five patients. Proper understanding of the biomechanics of different fracture patterns, assessment of bone quality, physiological needs of the patient and the capability of different implants available for surgical treatment, are essential for the selection of the surgical approach, type and fixation strategy. Ultimately, judicious planning is probably the most important factor influencing the outcome of treatment, in which fracture healing, maintenance of proper reduction and swift restoration of function are altogether the goals.

IntechOpen

2. Pathomechanics of distal femoral fractures

The most frequent mechanical complication of distal femoral fractures (DFF) is nonunion, reported in up to 19% of patients [3, 4]. Along with nonunion, varus collapse and hardware failure come together. This continues to occur despite advances in fracture fixation implants for this injury, reflecting the need for better understanding of different factors that influence the outcome. Modern implants include those advocated by the AO Foundation decades ago, such as the 95 degree blade-plate and the Dynamic Condylar Screw (DCS) [5–8]. Such devices are seldom used nowadays for acute fracture treatment. Being made of stainless steel, they provided strong fixation and resistance to fatigue, improving dramatically the quality of fixation and ultimately the results. However, their inherent stiffness was still a cause for atrophic nonunions (**Figure 1**). Advances in the knowledge of concepts such as stress and strain highlighted the importance of the mechanical environment in the process of bone healing [9–11]. Application of these concepts by the surgeon is the basis for the construction of biomechanically sound osteosynthesis, in which highly rigid constructs are being replaced by others allowing controlled micromotion, and subsequent stimulus for callus formation.

In more recent years, both anatomical, locked plates (LP), and retrograde interlocking intramedullary nails (RIMN) became the standard for operative management [4, 12]. Both types of fixation show similar rates of bone healing and functional outcome, despite dissimilarities. In some studies, intramedullary devices perform better than plates in terms of axial stiffness, whilst in others side plates were superior [13, 14]. Nonetheless, both methods are also associated with a high

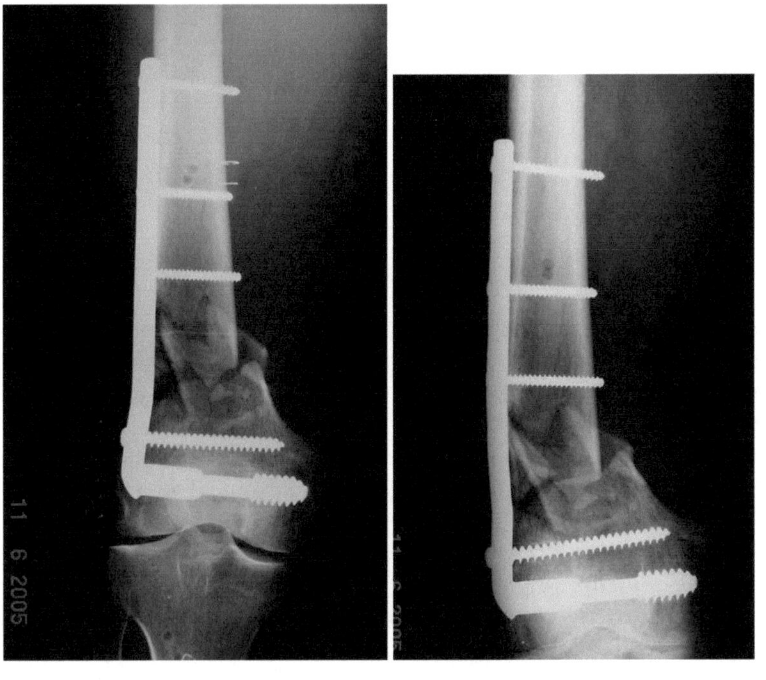

Figure 1.
Extraarticular distal femoral fracture, treated with a short Dynamic Condylar Screw (DCS). At follow up, nounion and failure in varus occurred. Metaphyseal comminution and a short side plate and working length are considerations to be taken into account to explain the result.

incidence of mechanical failures [4, 15–18]. Although having improved mechanical capabilities compared to previous implants, improper use, or unawareness of the importance of the balance between rigidity, stability and bone healing promotion, can lead to failure (**Figure 2**) [19].

Numerous in vitro reports have been published in recent years, showing improved mechanical capabilities with fixation techniques that combine lateral locking plates and medially placed additional plates, as well as the combination of lateral locking plates and locked intramedullary retrograde nails ("augmented RIMN") [20–25]. These studies report a significant increase in resistance to axial, rotational and bending forces, along with increased stiffness of such constructs, which has led to their application for clinical use, in pursuit of minimizing complications derived from implant failure. Several mechanical stress studies, as well as clinical studies, focus on fractures with bone defects and/or comminution, including fractures in osteoporotic patients, because they have high risk for failure. Ricci et al. published an analysis of the factors that may influence failure of fixation in distal femoral fractures, treated with laterally placed locked plates [26]. Various types of fractures were included: 64%

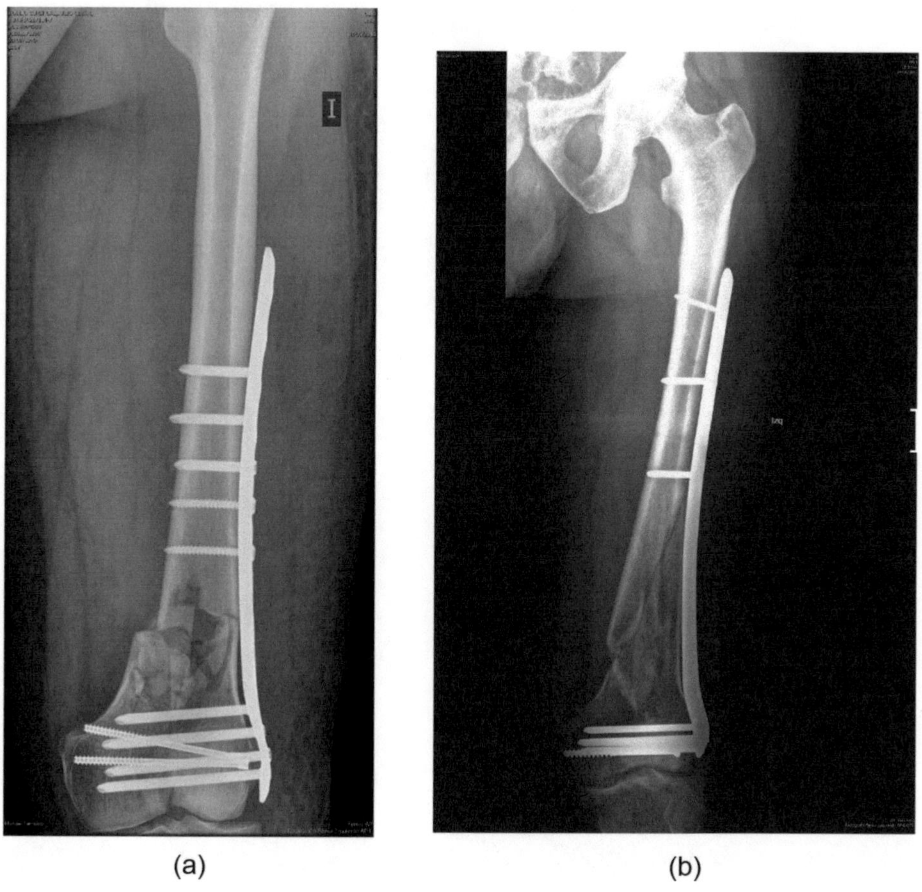

Figure 2.
(a) A3 closed fracture in a 50 year-old patient, treated with anatomical locking plate. AP x-ray at follow up shows atrophic nonunion. Selection of the length of the plate, together with the distribution of screws, may have played a role in the outcome. (b) Same fracture pattern in a 44 year-old patient, with more extended working length and less screw density. Uneventful consolidation has occurred after 6 months.

of 335 fractures were simple metaphyseal (A1 and A2), or simple articular (C1 or C2). They found that there were factors out of reach from the surgeon, such as severity of the injury (high energy, open fractures), young age (with more severe injuries), comorbidities such as diabetes, and smoking. Plate length, on the other hand, was also a contributing factor: shorter plates were associated with failures more frequently than long plates. The surgeon must therefore balance what is inherent to the fracture and the patient, with the available implants, elaborating a strategy that will ultimately lead to a construct design capable of minimizing the risk of failure.

In our opinion, DFF differ in the pathomechanical analysis that can be made whether they are simple extraarticular, comminuted extraarticular, or intraarticular, as well as if present in young or older (osteopenic) patients. Older patients with poor

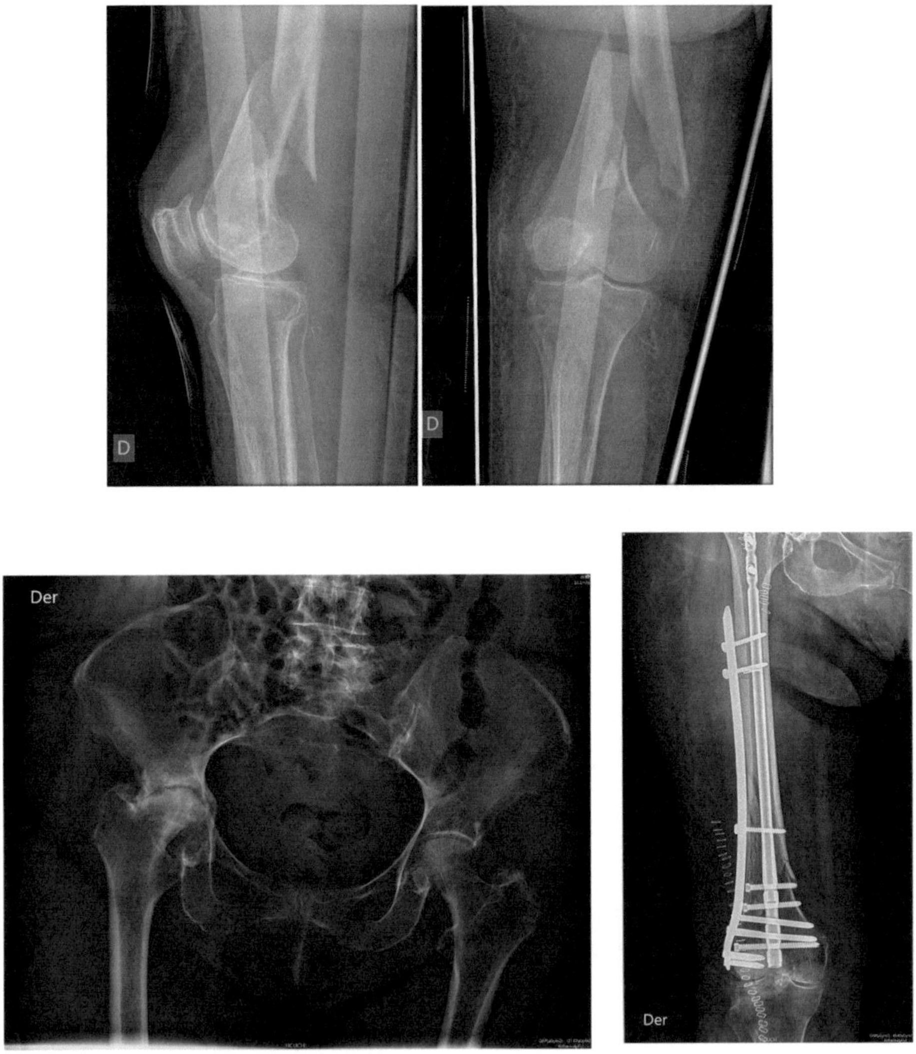

Figure 3.
Distal extraarticular fracture in a 75 year old patient with concomitant severe ipsilateral hip arthritis and rigidity. Despite absence of comminution, fixation was done with RIMN, augmented with a locking plate. This was decided in consideration of the age of the patient, and the incresed torsional stresses that the construct will withstand throughout the healing process, due to hip stifness.

DOI: http://dx.doi.org/10.5772/intechopen.110692

bone quality present inherent difficulties in obtaining stable internal fixation. There is data underlying the difficulties to accomplish "limited" weight-bearing in patients of advanced age, so it should be assumed that patients of a certain age will submit the construct to high forces from the early postoperative period [27, 28]. These considerations have decisive influence on the selection of the operative method.

Of note is the fact that advances in implant stability and rigidity may also present concerns about delayed healing. There is the need to balance the overall strength/stiffness of the construct and the appropriate micromotion that promotes callus formation. With patients of advanced age, however, the benefits of construct stability and endurance may outweigh the achievement of fracture healing, at least initially [28–31]. Postoperative compliance with controlled or "limited" weight bearing is very difficult to achieve in geriatric patients, as mentioned above. Therefore, implant stability and strength is of primary importance (**Figure 3**). These considerations do not apply, nonetheless, in the young patient with similar fractures. In this setting, promotion of bone healing is paramount for long term success and functional restoration. Therefore, careful and judicious application of any fixation method or technique should balance the maintenance of proper reduction while favoring bone healing, the latter by the means of providing a mechanical environment with adequate strain.

As aforementioned, a sound mechanical construct should take into consideration the quality of bone, the general status and age of the patient, and also the type of fracture. We consider it appropriate to analyze distal femoral fractures broadly distinguishing between those with and without articular involvement. Articular involvement has requirements for adequate fixation that differ from extraarticular fractures, whether comminuted or not. Anatomic articular reduction and rigid fixation is a principle that remains unchanged since first advocated by the AO [32]. This requires the use of individual screws for fragment fixation and articular restoration, which is most often followed by implantation of plates and/or intramedullary nails to unite the articular segment to the diaphysis. Within these two main categories, management decisions can be

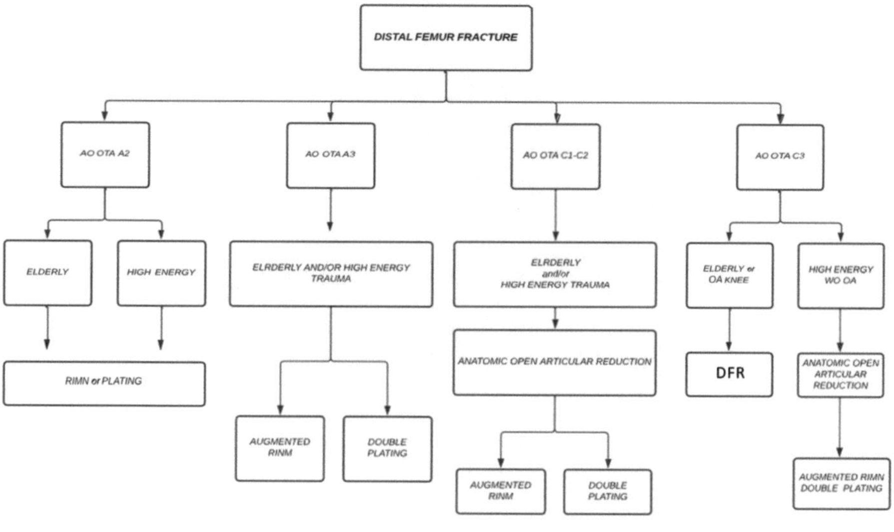

Figure 4.
Flowchart as a proposal for the management of distal femoral fractures. DFR: distal femoral replacement.

made when we include other components in the analysis (those inherent to the fracture and the patient) pertinent to the treatment plan. This could work as an algorithm for proper selection of surgical approach, implants and design of the construct (**Figure 4**).

3. Management of extraarticular fractures of the distal femur

Extraarticular fractures involving the metaphysis, and without comminution (type A1 and A2 fractures, according to AO/OTA), can be addressed efficiently with

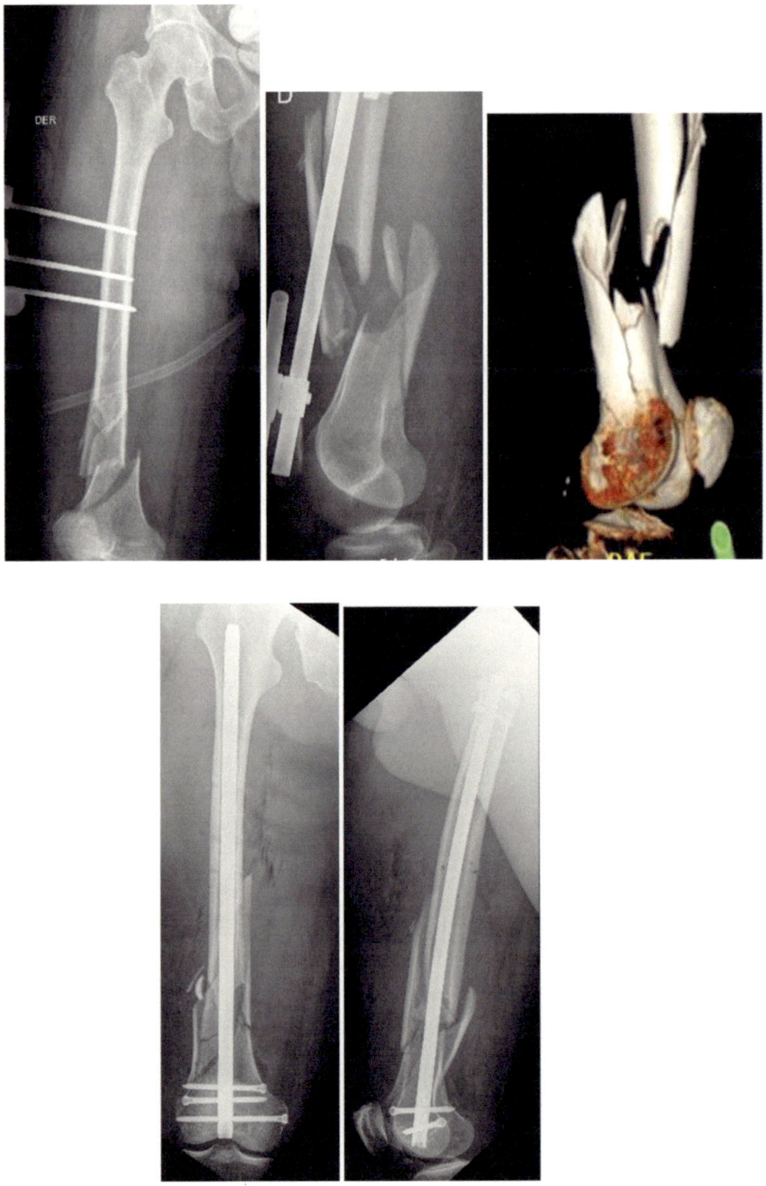

Figure 5.
Type A3 high-energy fracture, managed with RIMN and three distal locking screws.

either LP or RIMN (**Figure 5**) [33–37]. The presence of metaphyseal comminution and/or osteopenic bone involves a high risk of varus collapse and hardware failure [38] (type A3 fractures). For these fractures numerous biomechanical studies have been published, as mentioned before, in bone models with finite element analysis and in cadaver studies, in search for stronger fixation methods [38–41]. DeKeyser et al. reported a literature review on what has been investigated in terms of mechanical fixation of distal femoral fractures with a metaphyseal defect. As a summary, medial and lateral plate fixation (dual plating of the distal femur) and the combination of IMN and LP, showed greater strength and resistance to axial, torsional and bending forces, than conventional LP or INM fixation alone. Lodde et al. published a literature review on the clinical results of double plating, that included femoral shaft fractures in polytrauma patients, femoral nonunions, proximal femoral pathological fractures, periprosthetic fractures, and distal femoral fractures. They concluded that double plating is a valid alternative for management of the latter, with high union rates (88%), but also with a 33% complication rate. Steinberg et al. reported on clinical results in double plating for acute distal femoral fractures (intra and extraarticular), nonunions and periprosthetic fractures. Only one of 32 patients developed nonunion that required bone grafting, and one had a femoral shaft fracture proximal to the hardware, requiring lateral plate exchange. Bologna et al. published on a comparative cohort of patients treated either with single or double plating with C2 and C3 (AO-OTA) distal femoral and periprosthetic fractures. A statistically significant difference was found between the two groups in terms of nonunion and time to healing, in favor of dual plating. It is clear that increasing the strength and rigidity of the construct by adding a parallel medial plate has a correlation with better clinical results and fewer mechanical failures. However, there is still lack of definitive clinical evidence whether this augmentation -which leads to increased stiffness- ultimately allows proper bone healing. In cases of poor bone quality, a stronger construct may well withstand forces irrespective of fracture consolidation. It can be difficult to interpret and clearly define the presence of bone bridging in the fracture zone on plain X-rays. To our knowledge, no large scale study has been presented assessing bone healing with a more sensitive exam, such as multiplanar CT.

A few cases reporting on the advantages of the combination of LP- RIMN in fractures in osteopenic bone have been published, as well as femoral nonunions [29, 30, 42, 43]. It seems that this method allows for earlier weight bearing and functional recovery in older patients, due to the increased strength of the construct. Engaging both the plate and the nail with screws that interlock both implants may increase even further the resistance of the system.

In our experience, the combination of IMN and LP ("augmented RIMN") in the management of fractures with metaphyseal comminution results in a construct which combines the benefits of both implants (**Figure 6**). It has been argued that it results in a more even distribution of forces, which allow for earlier weight bearing, while minimizing the risk of hardware failure [29, 44]. From the mechanical standpoint, a long lateral locking plate with far-proximal cortical screws tangential to the nail, provides a longer working length and higher resistance to cantilever forces towards varus at the proximal end of the plate (which is acting as a true tension band), in an attempt to minimize proximal screw loosening and pull-out (**Figure 7**). In our initial experience with shorter plates, however, toggling and loosening of these screws was not followed by progressive deformity in varus. We believe that the presence of a long, locked intramedullary device helps in maintaining alignment.

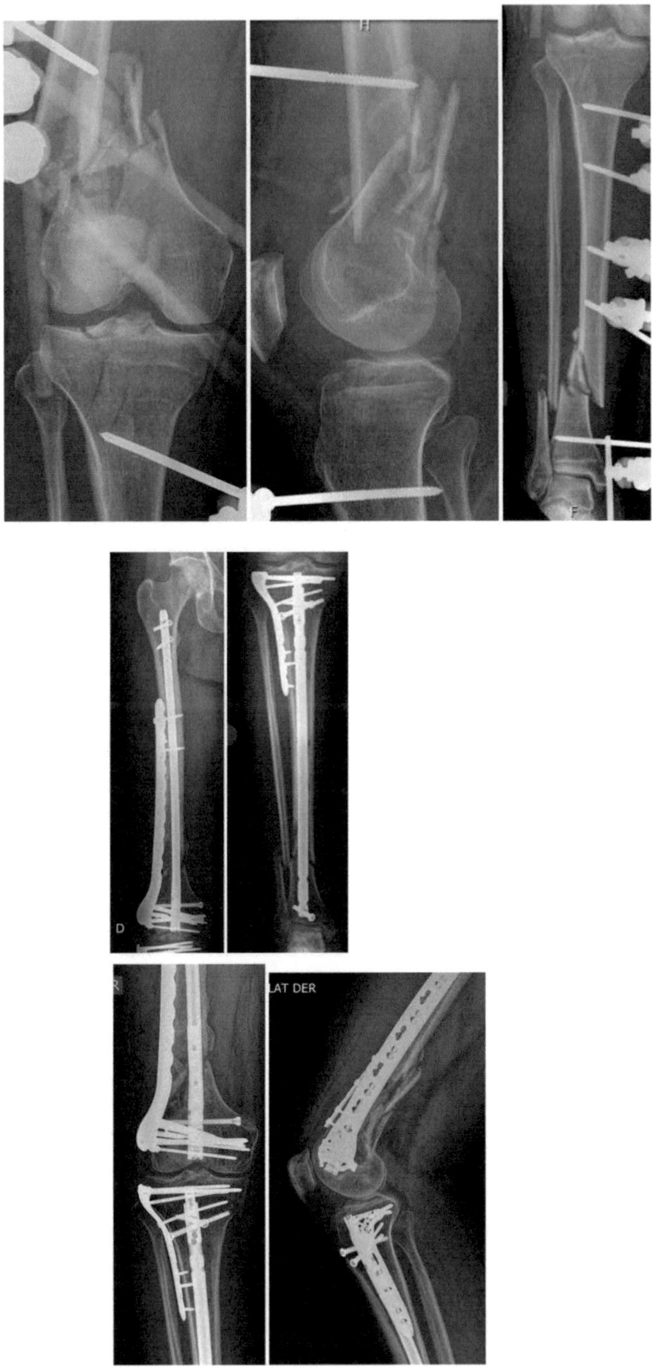

Figure 6.
High-energy floating knee injury (Fraser type IIC), with open segmental tibial fracture. After damage-control orthopaedic management, definitive fixation was performed with a nail and plate combination for the femur and tibia. Reduction of the articular femoral fracture was done with 3.5 mm. cortical screws, and additional 3.5 mm. one-third tubular plate. No other procedures were needed until healing.

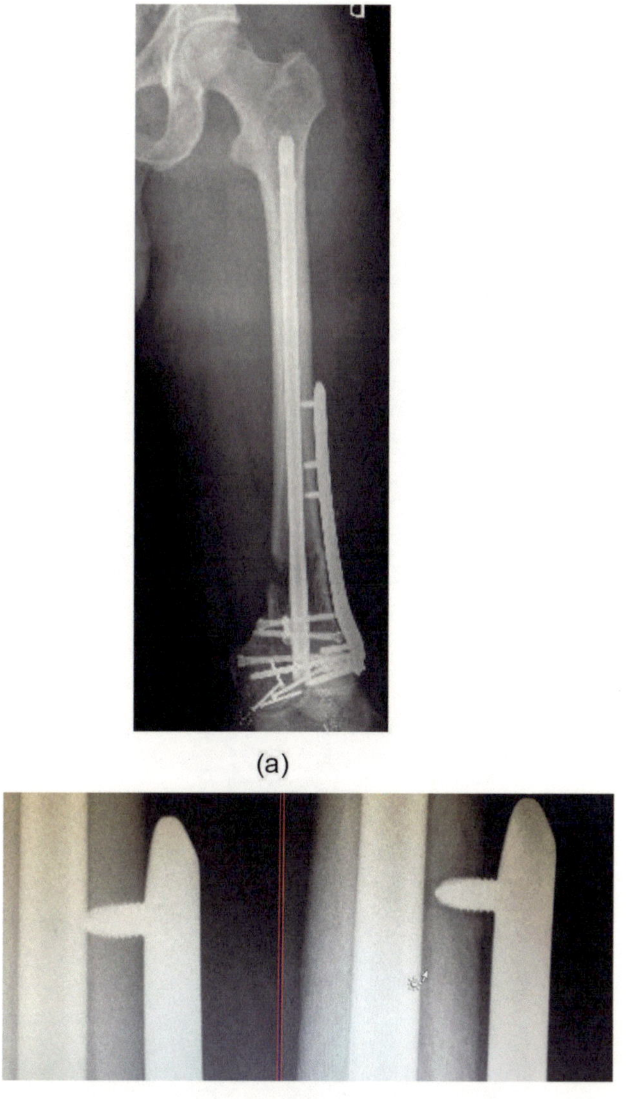

(a)

(b)

Figure 7.
(a) AP X-ray showing fixation of a A3 distal femoral fracture with nail and plate combination. A short lateral locking plate and proximal monocortical locked screws were used. (b) After 5 months, loosening of most proximal locked screw is seen, due to toggling. To prevent this, extended length of the plate proximally, and proximal bicortical screws, would have been appropriate.

Recent advances in design have brought into market extraosseous devices that engage to a RIMN through screws, adding significant stability to conventional nail interlocking screws [45]. This locked "washer" gets "unitized" to the intramedullary nail, which in mechanical testing -together with still limited clinical experience- has shown significant improvement in endurance and strength. The combination of RIMN plus a lateral locking plate acts using the same principle. This "washer",

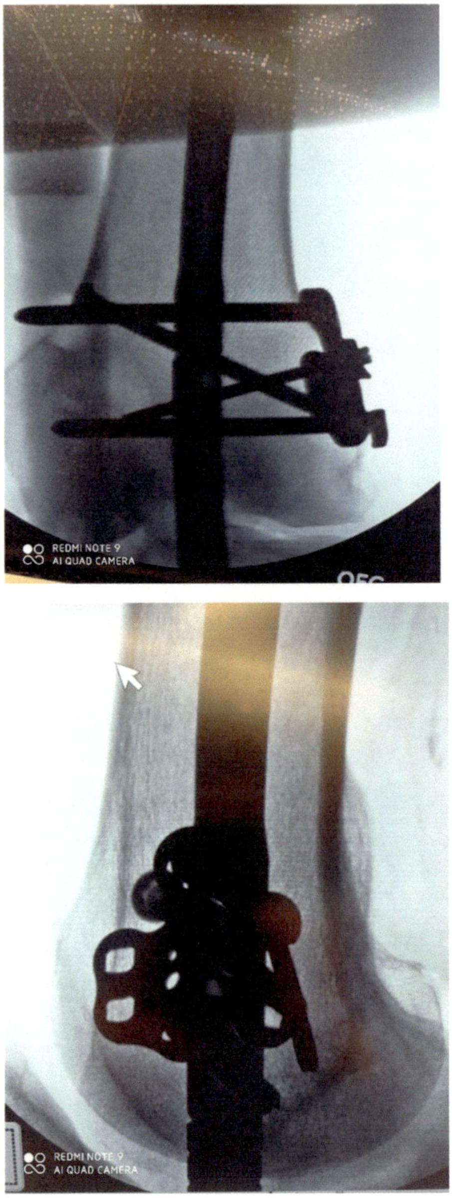

Figure 8.
AP and lateral view of the "locking washer" in place, which engages two locking holes of a retrograde nail with screws that are locked to the external device, providing significant increase in stability over interlocking screws alone.

moreover, could have the additional advantage of avoiding submuscular dissection for placing a long lateral plate (**Figure 8**).

4. Management of intraarticular fractures

Articular involvement should be addressed with anatomical restoration of the joint as a prime objective. Open reduction is often required. Additional fixation of the articular segment to the femoral diaphysis can be achieved by different methods, either "minimally invasive" or open. As mentioned previously, considerations for the planning of the approach and the selection of implants shall consider the amount of fracture comminution, the quality of the bone, the age and physiological needs of the patient, and -for articular fractures- whether there is previous joint arthritis.

Currently, with modern RIMN and anatomical locking plates, either simple or complex articular fractures can be properly managed in terms of initial fixation and alignment (**Figure 9**) [46–50]. However, comminuted articular fractures -as well as those with metaphyseal comminution, as mentioned before-, together with other specific fracture patterns, have been associated with a high rate of nounion and hardware failure [15, 26, 51, 52]. Recently, Nino et al. published on 16 patients with articular comminution, that were treated with articular screw fixation and RIMN, with a high degree of success in terms of fracture healing, without the need of additional procedures to promote union [53]. However, 38% of patients had a complication, most commonly knee stiffness. To minimize the risk of fixation failure and nonunion in cases of comminution and/or poor bone quality, and as mentioned before, the advent of techniques such as coupling intramedullary devices to laterally placed plates or locked "washers", as well as the addition of medial plates as a supporting medial strut, have come into play, with clinical evidence supporting their use (**Figure 10**).

Articular involvement—even with comminution—is not an impediment for the use of RIMN. Proper articular reduction and fixation can be undertaken with small-diameter screws (2.7 or 3.5 mm. cortical screws), which provide sound fixation of articular fragments, and leave space for the insertion of a nail. RIMN becomes a supporting column placed in the mechanical axis of the femur, therefore resisting axial and bending forces, acting as a load-sharing device. "Augmentation", by the addition of a lateral locking plate—or an interlocking "washer"—adds significant resistance to mechanical failure, with a higher endurance of the construct until bone healing occurs.

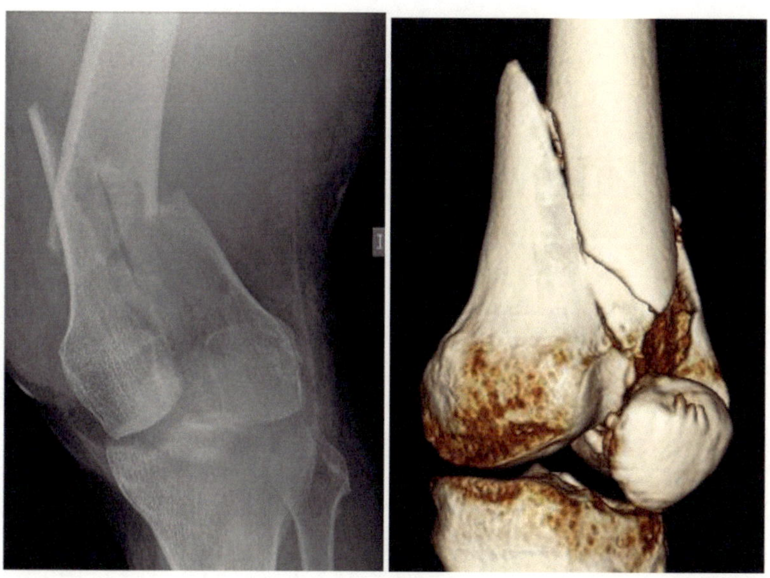

Figure 9.
C1 fracture, treated with open parapatellar approach, reduction and fixation of the condyles with 3.5 mm. cortical screws, and RIMN as definitive fixation. Callus formation and healing is seen after 6 months.

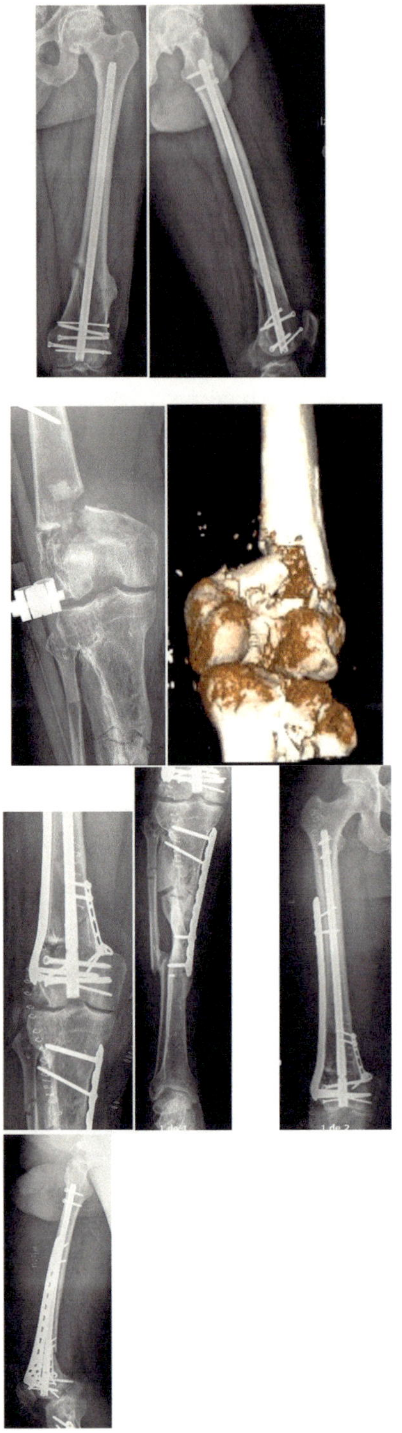

Figure 10.
High-energy floating knee (Fraser type IIB) in a patient with a previously healed tibial fracture, and an osteoarticular defect of the lateral femoral condyle, due to trauma 9 years before the actual scenario. The articular distal femoral fracture was managed with 3.5 mm. cortical screws, and a 3.5 mm. wrist T plate for reduction to the diaphysis, followed by nail and plate combination. The tibial fracture was fixed with a percutaneous plate, due to absence of displacement, and because the tibial canal was assumed to be occluded by the previous fracture.

The presence of joint arthritis, especially in older patients, should be a main consideration when planning surgical treatment. In such patients, distal femoral replacement with a distal femoral megaprosthesis and a rotating hinge, has been advocated as an excellent treatment method, allowing for swift functional recovery [54–58]. Internal fixation—whichever the method—is subjected to high rotational and bending forces due to joint stiffness, which is often aggravated by poor bone quality, as well as the difficulty (as previously mentioned) in restricting function postoperatively in order to decrease the risk of hardware failure. In addition, older patients with distal femoral fractures share similar epidemiological characteristics with those having proximal femoral fractures, including mortality rates [59], so

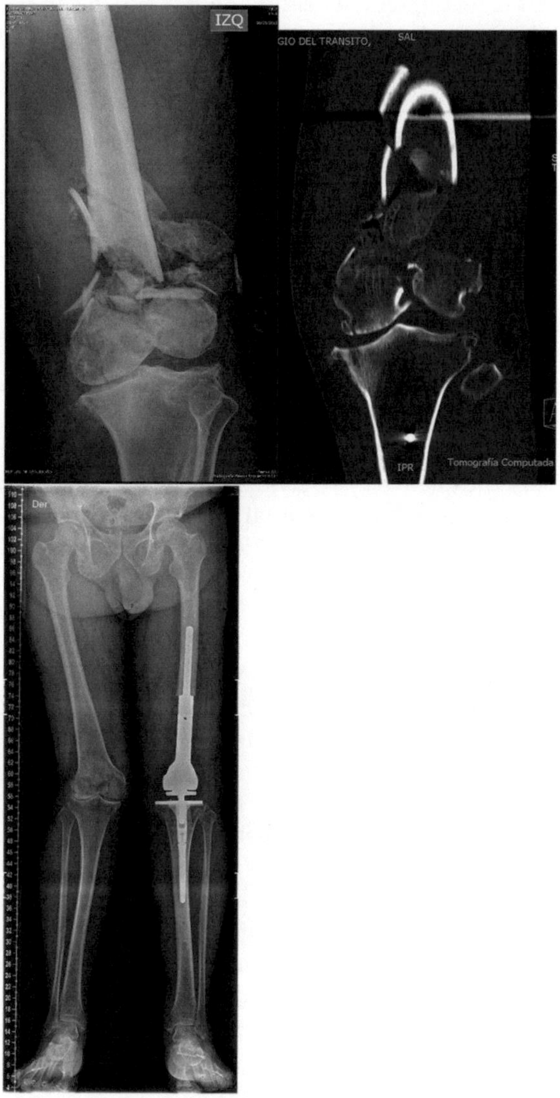

Figure 11.
C3 distal femoral fracture in a 70 year-old patient. X-rays and CT show extensive articular comminution, and signs of knee arthritis. A resection of the distal femur and reconstruction with a modular tumor endoprosthesis and rotating hinge was done. Swift postoperative recovery and return to funtion was possible.

considerations for operative treatment and early return to function should be the same As such, primary treatment with distal femoral resection and replacement by a rotating hinged prosthetic knee is a very valuable alternative (**Figure 11**). Aside from the aforementioned advantages, complications or re-interventions in distal femoral replacements are not higher than those reported with fracture fixation techniques.

5. Essentials of surgical technique

Our preference for all cases requiring internal fixation, is positioning in supine. A sterile and discardable torniquet is a useful adjunct which can be used to facilitate exposure, and can be later removed if needed, so it does not interfere with insertion of plates and/or retrograde nails. Whenever RIMN becomes part of the fixation method, we advocate the use of long nails, extending proximally to the metaphysis, in between the two trochanters. This may provide protection of the entire bone segment, therefore minimizing the risk of periprosthetic fractures.

If open reduction is indicated, whether the fracture is intraarticular or extraarticular, we have progressively shifted our choice to a lateral para-quadricipital approach. It was originally described as a trans-articular approach for fracture fixation with plates [60]. This allows excellent exposure of both femoral condyles, facilitating direct visualization and reduction of articular fragments, if present. Deep flexion of the knee allows for the whole contour of the articular surface to be assessed. At times, in cases of metaphyseal comminution (A3 or C2/C3 fractures), this approach allows the surgeon to directly reduce the condyles to the diaphysis, and use small plates or K wires for provisional fixation. Access to the femoral diaphysis can be undertaken by dividing longitudinally the quadriceps between the rectus anterior and vastus lateralis very proximally, to expose the intact proximal diaphysis. Direct assessment -and/or indirect assessment with fluoroscopy- of overall alignment can be done. The same approach allows for placement of a lateral locking plate onto the condyles, which is then slid proximally in a closed manner, to be finally attached to the proximal diaphysis with percutaneous screws.

For the combined use of RIMN and locking plates ("augmented RIMN"), and depending on the details of the fracture pattern as seen during exposure, at times the first implant to be used is the plate, which is fixed to bone with short (usually 30 or 32 mm long) locking screws distally and monocortical (14 mm long) locked screws to the diaphysis (**Figure 12**), in order to allow unobstructed insertion of a RIMN. Whenever possible, we attempt to have at least one locking screw inserted from the plate engaging one of the interlocking holes of the nail. This results in a much stronger construct distally. We should outline that, at the end of the procedure, and in light that proximal monocortical screws might toggle and loosen due to repetitive cantilever forces towards varus, the two most proximal screws in the plate are replaced with bicortical 4.5 large fragment screws. These usually have a trajectory tangential to the intramedullary nail, which enhances their resistance to pull out. Closure of the longitudinal quadriceps split is done with non-absorbable suture in order to restore continuity of the muscular unit, and to allow prompt full passive range of motion and active isometric muscle contraction.

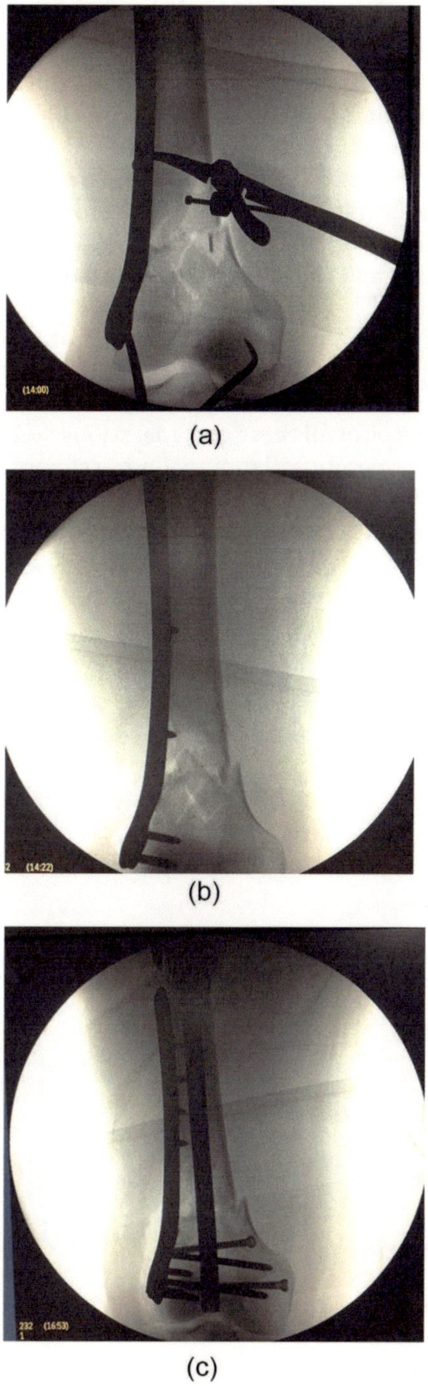

Figure 12.
(a–c) Direct approach and reduction of the fracture by means of a lateral locking plate. Monocortical locked screws proximally and 30 mm-long locked screws distally were used for reduction and provisional fixation, allowing unobstructed insertion of a RIMN.

6. Summary

Distal femoral fracture management illustrates the evolution in the treatment of fractures that have significant impact on function and quality of life. New developments in fixation techniques, together with an increased understanding of the influence of mechanics in the process of fracture healing (the balance between stress and strain) has led to constant evolution in the design and selection of implants for these injuries (and combination of implants when needed). Together with a careful evaluation of the fracture pattern and the condition of the patient, the surgeon can wisely plan the best fixation method.

Distal femoral fractures, whether extra or intraarticular, with or without comminution, presenting in young, active patients (high-energy fractures and/or polytrauma) or in older patients with osteoporosis and/or knee arthritis, should be evaluated taking into account all these considerations. Selection of the surgical approach is also part of preoperative planning. Our preference for anterior, paraquadricipital approach is based on the excellent visualization of femoral condyles, metaphyseal area and proximal femoral diaphysis. In addition, it does not impede standard submuscular sliding of a lateral plate proximally and percutaneous screw fixation. Availability of diverse implants, experience of the surgical team, and dedicated, multidisciplinary care for appropriate postoperative rehabilitation, are additional important factors for successful treatment of these complex injuries.

Author details

Luis Bahamonde[1,2,3*] and Alvaro Zamorano[1,3]

1 Hospital Mutual de Seguridad, Chile

2 Clinica Las Condes, Santiago, Chile

3 University of Chile, Santiago, Chile

*Address all correspondence to: lbahamondemunoz@gmail.com

References

[1] Elsoe R, Ceccotti A, Larsen P. Population-based epidemiology and incidence of distal femur fractures. International Orthopaedics. 2018;**42**:191-196

[2] Pietu G, Lebaron M, Flecher X, et al. Epidemiology of distal femur fractures in France in 2011-12. Orthopaedics & Traumatology, Surgery & Research. 2014;**100**:545-548

[3] Ebraheim N, Martin BS, Sochacki K, Liu J. Nonunion of distal femoral fractures: A systematic review. Orthopaedic Surgery. 2013;**5**:46-50

[4] Koso RE, Terhoeve C, Steen RG, Zura R. Healing, nonunion, and re-operation after internal fixation of diaphyseal and distal femoral fractures: A systematic review and meta-analysis. International Orthopaedics. 2018;**42**(11):2675-2683

[5] Radford P, Howell C. The AO dynamic condylar screw for fractures of the femur. Injury. 1992;**23**:89-93

[6] Vallier H, Immler W. Comparison of the 95-degree angled blade plate and the locking condylar plate for the treatment of distal femoral fractures. Journal of Orthopaedic Trauma. 2012;**26**(6):327-332

[7] Heiney JP, Barnett MD, Vrabec GA, Schoenfeld AJ, Baji A, Njus GO. Distal femoral fixation: A biomechanical comparison of trigen retrograde intramedullary (i.m.) nail, dynamic condylar screw (DCS), and locking compression plate (LCP) condylar plate. The Journal of Trauma. 2009;**66**(2):443-449

[8] Merchan E, Maestu P, Blanco R. Blade-plating of closed displaced supracondylar fractures of the distal femur with the AO system. The Journal of Trauma. 1992;**32**(2):174-178

[9] Elliott DS, Newman KJH, Forward DP, Hahn DM, Ollivere B, Kojima K, et al. A unified theory of bone healing and nonunion: BHN theory. The Bone & Joint Journal. 2016;**98**(7):884-891

[10] Glatt V, Evans CH, Tetsworth K. A concert between biology and biomechanics: The influence of the mechanical environment on bone healing. Frontiers in Physiology. 2017;**7**:1-18

[11] Perren SM. Fracture healing. Osteosynthesis in the Hand: Current Concepts: FESSH Instructional Course. 2008;**2008**:4-11

[12] Hake ME, Davis ME, Perdue AM, Goulet JA. Modern implant options for the treatment of distal femur fractures. JAAOS-Journal of the American Academy of Orthopaedic Surgeons. 2019;**27**(19):e867-e875

[13] Wähnert D, Hoffmeier K, Fröber R, Hofmann GO, Mückley T. Distal femur fractures of the elderly—Different treatment options in a biomechanical comparison. Injury. 2011;**42**(7):655-659

[14] Meyer RW, Plaxton NA, Postak PD, Gilmore A, Froimson MI, Greenwald AS. Mechanical comparison of a distal femoral side plate and a retrograde intramedullary nail. Journal of Orthopaedic Trauma. 2000;**14**(6):398-404

[15] Peschiera V, Staletti L, Cavanna M, Saporito M, Berlusconi M. Predicting the failure in distal femur fractures. Injury. 2018;**49**:S2-S7

[16] Henderson CE, Kuhl LL, Fitzpatrick DC, Marsh JI. Locking plates

for distal femur fractures: Is there a problem with fracture healing? Journal of Orthopaedic Trauma. 2011;**25**:S8-S14

[17] Papadokostakis G, Papakostidis C, Dimitriou R, Giannoudis PV. The role and efficacy of retrograding nailing for the treatment of diaphyseal and distal femoral fractures: A systematic review of the literature. Injury. 2005;**36**(7):813-822

[18] Hoffmann MF, Jones CB, Sietsema DL, Tornetta P, Koenig SJ. Clinical outcomes of locked plating of distal femoral fractures in a retrospective cohort. Journal of Orthopaedic Surgery and Research. 2013;**8**(1):1-9

[19] Harvin WH, Oladeji LO, Della Rocca GJ, Murtha YM, Volgas DA, Stannard JP, et al. Working length and proximal screw constructs in plate osteosynthesis of distal femur fractures. Injury. 2017;**48**(11):2597-2601

[20] Goodnough LH, Salazar BP, Chen MJ, Storaci H, Guzman R, Heffner M, et al. Supplemental medial small fragment fixation adds stability to distal femur fixation: A biomechanical study. Injury. 2021;**52**(7):1670-1672

[21] DeKeyser GJ, Hakim AJ, O'Neill DC, Schlickewei CW, Marchand LS, Haller JM. Biomechanical and anatomical considerations for dual plating of distal femur fractures: A systematic literature review. Archives of Orthopaedic and Trauma Surgery. 2021;**2021**:1-13

[22] Fontenot PB, Diaz M, Stoops K, Barrick B, Santoni B, Mir H. Supplementation of lateral locked plating for distal femur fractures: A biomechanical study. Journal of Orthopaedic Trauma. 2019;**33**(12):642-648

[23] Başci O, Karakaşli A, Kumtepe E, et al. Combination of anatomical locking plate and retrograde intramedullary nail in distal femoral fractures: Comparison of mechanical stability. Eklem Hast Cerrahisi. 2015;**26**:21-26

[24] Park KH, Oh CW, Park IH, Kim JW, Lee JH, Kim HJ. Additional fixation of medial plate over the unstable lateral locked plating of distal femur fractures: A biomechanical study. Injury. 2019;**50**(10):1593-1598

[25] Wright DJ, DeSanto DJ, McGarry MH, Lee TQ, Scolaro JA. Supplemental fixation of supracondylar distal femur fractures: A biomechanical comparison of dual-plate and plate-nail constructs. Journal of Orthopaedic Trauma. 2020;**34**(8):434-440

[26] Ricci WM, Streubel PN, Morshed S, Collinge CA, Nork SE, Gardner MJ. Risk factors for failure of locked plate fixation of distal femur fractures: An analysis of 335 cases. Journal of Orthopaedic Trauma. 2014;**28**(2):83-89

[27] Canton G, Giraldi G, Dussi M, Ratti C, Murena L. Osteoporotic distal femur fractures in the elderly: peculiarities and treatment strategies. Acta Bio Medica. 2019;**90**(Suppl. 12):25

[28] Von Rüden C, Augat P. Failure of fracture fixation in osteoporotic bone. Injury. 2016;**47**:S3-S10

[29] Liporace FA, Yoon RS. Nail plate combination technique for native and periprosthetic distal femur fractures. Journal of Orthopaedic Trauma. 2019;**33**(2):e64-e68

[30] Garala K, Ramoutar D, Li J, Syed F, Arastu M, Ward J, et al. Distal femoral fractures: A comparison between single lateral plate fixation and a combined femoral nail and plate fixation. Injury. 2022;**53**(2):634-639

[31] Kammerlander P, Riedmaller P, Gosch M, Zegg M, Kammerlander-

Knauer U, Schmid R, et al. Functional outcome and mortality in geriatric distal femoral fractures. Injury. 2012;**43**:1096-1110

[32] Müller ME, Perren SM, Allgöwer M, Müller ME, Schneider R, Willenegger H. Manual of Internal Fixation: Techniques Recommended by the AO-ASIF Group. Springer Science & Business Media; 1991

[33] Ehlinger M, Ducrot G, Adam P, Bonnomet F. Distal femur fractures. Surgical techniques and a review of the literature. Orthopaedics & Traumatology: Surgery & Research. 2013;**99**(3):353-360

[34] von Keudell A, Shoji K, Nasr M, Lucas R, Dolan R, Weaver MJ. Treatment options for distal femur fractures. Journal of Orthopaedic Trauma. 2016;**30**:S25-S27

[35] Gangavalli AK, Nwachuku CO. Management of distal femur fractures in adults: An overview of options. Orthopedic Clinics. 2016;**47**(1):85-96

[36] Beltran MJ, Gary JL, Collinge CA. Management of distal femur fractures with modern plates and nails: State of the art. Journal of Orthopaedic Trauma. 2015;**29**(4):165-172

[37] Wilson JL, Squires M, McHugh M, Ahn J, Perdue A, Hake M. The geriatric distal femur fracture: Nail, plate or both? European Journal of Orthopaedic Surgery & Traumatology. 2022:1-9

[38] Tahami M, Vaziri AS, Tahmasebi MN, Vosoughi F, Khalilizad M, Shakiba S, et al. Practical approach to the native distal femur fractures in the elderly: A rapid review over the recent trends. Injury. 2022;**53**:2389-2394

[39] Zhang W, Li J, Zhang H, Wang M, Li L, Zhou J, et al. Biomechanical assessment of single LISS versus double-plate osteosynthesis in the AO type 33-C2 fractures: A finite element analysis. Injury. 2018;**49**:2142-2146

[40] Lodde MF, Raschke MJ, Stolberg-Stolberg J, Everding J, Rosslenbroich S, Katthagen JC. Union rates and functional outcome of double plating of the femur: Systematic review of the literature. Archives of Orthopaedic and Trauma Surgery. 2022;**142**(6):1009-1030

[41] Steinberg EL, Elis J, Steinberg Y, Salai M, Ben-Tov T. A double-plating approach to distal femur fracture: A clinical study. Injury. 2017;**48**(10):2260-2265

[42] Kontakis MG, Giannoudis PV. Nail plate combination in fractures of the distal femur in the elderly: A new paradigm for optimum fixation and early mobilization? Injury. Feb 2022;**54**(2):288-291. DOI: 10.1016/j.injury.2022.11.035

[43] Attum B, Douleh D, Whiting PS, White-Dzuro GA, Dodd AC, Shen MS, et al. Outcomes of distal femur nonunions treated with a combined nail/plate construct and autogenous bone grafting. Journal of Orthopaedic Trauma. 2017;**31**(9):e301-e304

[44] Liporace FA, Aneja A, Carroll EA, Yoon RS. Maintaining the neutral axis in the treatment of distal femur fractures via dual plate or nail plate combination technique: When and how? Journal of Orthopaedic Trauma. 2021;**35**:S38-S40

[45] Liporace FA, Tang A, Jankowski JM, Yoon RS. Distal femur: Nail plate combination and the linked construct. OTA International. 2022;**5**(3):e172

[46] Gwathmey WF, Jones-Quaidoo SM, Kahler D, Hurwitz S, Cui Q. Distal

femoral fractures: Current concepts. JAAOS-Journal of the American Academy of Orthopaedic Surgeons. 2010;**18**(10):597-607

[47] Piétu G, Ehlinger M. Minimally invasive internal fixation of distal femur fractures. Orthopaedics & Traumatology: Surgery & Research. 2017;**103**(1):S161-S169

[48] Ristevski B, Nauth A, Williams DS, Hall JA, Whelan DB, Bhandari M, et al. Systematic review of the treatment of periprosthetic distal femur fractures. Journal of Orthopaedic Trauma. 2015;**28**(5):307-312

[49] Zlowodzki M, Bhandari M, Marek DJ, Cole PA, Kregor PJ. Operative treatment of acute distal femur fractures: Systematic review of 2 comparative studies and 45 case series (1989 to 2005). Journal of Orthopaedic Trauma. 2006;**20**(5):366-371

[50] Virk JS, Garg SK, Gupta P, Jangira V, Singh J, Rana S. Distal femur locking plate: The answer to all distal femoral fractures. Journal of Clinical and Diagnostic Research: JCDR. 2016;**10**(10):RC01

[51] Hsu C, Yang J, Yeh T, Shen H, Pan R, Wu C. Early fixation failure of locked plating in complex distal femoral fractures: Root causes analysis. Formosan Medical Association Journal. 2021;**120**:395-403

[52] Lupescu O, Nagea M, Patru C, Vasilache C, Popescu GI. Treatment options for distal femoral fractures. Maedica. 2015;**10**(2):117

[53] Nino S, Parry JA, Avilucea FR, Haidukewych GJ, Langford JR. Retrograde intramedullary nailing of comminuted intra-articular distal femur fractures results in high union rate. European Journal of Orthopaedic Surgery & Traumatology. 2022;**32**(8):1577-1582

[54] Bell KM, Johnstone AJ, Court-Brown CM, Hughes SP. Primary knee arthroplasty for distal femoral fractures in elderly patients. The Journal of Bone and Joint Surgery. 1992;**74**(3):400-402

[55] Bettin CC, Weinlein JC, Toy PC, Heck RK. Distal femoral replacement for acute distal femoral fractures in elderly patients. Journal of Orthopaedic Trauma. 2016;**30**(9):503-509

[56] Rosen AL, Strauss E. Primary total knee arthroplasty for complex distal femur fractures in elderly patients. Clinical Orthopaedics and Related Research. 2004;**425**:101-105

[57] Hart GP, Kneisl JS, Springer BD, Patt JC, Karunakar MA. Open reduction vs distal femoral replacement arthroplasty for comminuted distal femur fractures in the patients 70 years and older. The Journal of Arthroplasty. 2017;**32**:202-206

[58] Meluzio MC, Oliva MS, Minutillo F, Ziranu A, Saccomanno MF, Maccauro G. The use of knee mega-prosthesis for the management of distal femoral fractures: A systematic review. Injury. 2020;**51**:S17-S22

[59] Smith JR, Halliday R, Aquilina AL, Morrison RJ, Yip GC, McArthur J. Distal femoral fractures: The need to review the standard of care. Injury. 2015;**46**(6):1084-1088

[60] Krettek C, Miclau T, Stephan C, Tscheme H. Transarticular approach and retrograde plate osteosynthesis (TARPO): An alternative surgical approach for complex distal intra-articular femur fractures. Techniques in Orthopaedics. 1999;**14**(3):219-229

Chapter 5

Calcaneus Fractures

McKenna W. Box, Grayson A. Domingue, Neil J. Werthmann, Jan P. Szatkowski and John T. Riehl

Abstract

The calcaneus is the most frequently fractured tarsal bone, making up 60% of all adult tarsal fractures. While many calcaneus fractures can be managed nonoperatively, operative management of displaced, intra-articular fractures can prevent long-term deformity and may result in improved outcomes compared to nonoperative management. Three of the most common surgical treatment options are open reduction internal fixation, closed reduction with percutaneous pinning, and primary subtalar arthrodesis. This chapter reviews the epidemiology, relevant anatomy, biomechanics, clinical presentation, diagnosis, and management of calcaneus fractures.

Keywords: calcaneus, Sanders classification, sinus tarsi approach, external fixation, hindfoot fracture, heel fracture, extensile lateral approach

1. Introduction

Calcaneus fractures are the most common fracture of the tarsal bones, comprising 60% of all adult tarsal fractures [1]. The incidence of calcaneus fractures is 11.5 per 100,000 annually and occurs 2.4 times more in males than in females [2, 3]. The peak incidence for males occurs between 20 and 29 years, while for females, incidence peaks between 60 and 70 years of age [3, 4].

Calcaneus fractures are commonly present in younger populations due to a fall from a height [5, 6]. In osteoporotic individuals, the strong contraction of the gastrocsoleus complex through the Achilles tendon can cause calcaneal tuberosity fractures. Almost 77% of calcaneus fractures have associated injuries, highlighting the importance of a thorough evaluation for associated occult fractures in calcaneus fractures [7].

2. Anatomy

Understanding the anatomy and articulations of the calcaneus is crucial for diagnosing and treating calcaneus fractures (**Figure 1**) [8, 9]. The unique three-dimensional shape can make evaluation and conceptualization of surgical techniques difficult for the novice. The superior calcaneal surface contains three facets. The posterior, middle/sustentacular, and anterior facets articulate with the talus's anterior, middle, and posterior articular surfaces, forming the talocalcaneal (or subtalar) joint. The larger posterior facet of the calcaneus is convex, articulating with the talus above. The posterior facet is the major weight-bearing surface of the calcaneus. Due to the

IntechOpen

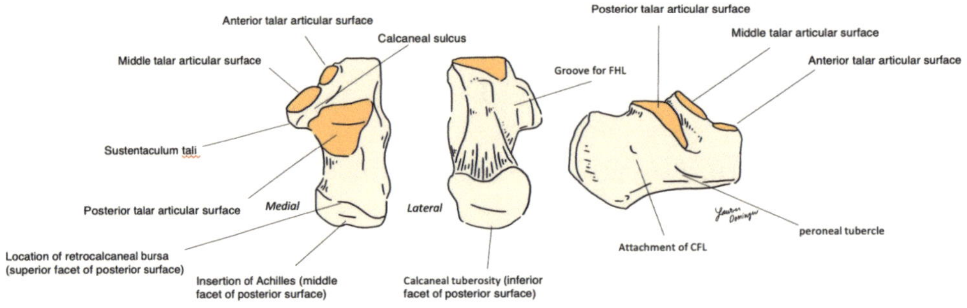

Figure 1.
Anatomic landmarks of the calcaneus.

high loads placed through the posterior facet, calcaneus fractures from axial loading often cause articular fragmentation. Anatomic reduction and fixation of the posterior facet are paramount to reducing the incidence of post-traumatic arthritis [10]. The calcaneus's smaller anterior and middle facets are concave in shape and separated from the posterior facet by the interosseous calcaneal ligament. However, a wide range of anatomical variations in the anterior and middle facets have been reported, ranging from a single ovoid-shaped facet to completely separated facets [11]. The middle facet lies on the superior surface of the sustentaculum tali. A posteromedial-directed groove called the calcaneal sulcus runs between the posterior and middle facets. A corresponding groove on the talus, called the sulcus tali, also runs between the posterior and middle facets of the talus. Together, these grooves make up the talo-calcaneal joint articulation and form the sinus tarsi (tarsal sinus/talocalcaneal sulcus) between the sulcus tali and calcaneal sulcus. Within the sinus tarsi lies an anastomosis between the peroneal and posterior tibial arteries and the cutaneous dorsolateral nerve of the superficial peroneal nerve [12]. Five ligaments are also contained in the sinus tarsi, the interosseous talocalcaneal ligament, the cervical ligament, and the medial, intermediate, and lateral root of the inferior extensor retinaculum. The primary function of these ligaments is to stabilize the talocalcaneal joint.

The medial surface of the calcaneus contains the sustentaculum tali (A.K.A. constant fragment). Superiorly, it sits against the middle talar articular facet. Inferiorly, this surface contains the groove for the flexor hallucis longus (FHL) tendon. The sustentaculum tali is bound to the talus by the interosseous talocalcaneal ligaments, spring ligament, and deltoid ligament. Fractures through the sustentaculum tali are rare and highly associated with intra-articular calcaneus fractures [13–15]. Due to the ligamentous connections on the sustentaculum tali, fractures are commonly nondisplaced [16], earning this portion of the calcaneus the term "constant fragment".

The lateral surface of the calcaneus has a bony prominence known as the peroneal tubercle. This structure lies in close relation to the tendons of the peroneus brevis and peroneus longus. The peroneus brevis passes anterior to the peroneal tubercle, and the peroneus longus travels inferior to it. The calcaneofibular ligament attaches proximally to the peroneal tubercle.

The posterior (nonarticular) surface of the calcaneus has three facets. The superior facet contains the retrocalcaneal bursa. The middle facet serves as the attachment for the Achilles tendon. The inferior facet forms the calcaneal tuberosity [17]. The anterior surface of the calcaneus contains the articular facet for the calcaneocuboid joint and the bifurcate ligament, which attaches the calcaneus to the cuboid and navicular.

3. Biomechanics

The calcaneus provides important static and dynamic functions of the foot and ankle. At rest, the static arch of the foot places 60% of weight-bearing stress on the plantar aponeurosis [18]. The plantar aponeurosis can absorb more stress as it becomes tauter, known as the windlass effect [19]. The windlass effect is essentially the tightening of the plantar fascia with dorsiflexion of the metatarsophalangeal joint, which elevates the medial longitudinal arch. The calcaneus's shape allows the plantar aponeurosis to change tension without collapsing the lateral or medial longitudinal arches [19]. The calcaneus dynamically supports movement and function with inversion and eversion through the subtalar joint, forming a rigid lever arm during toe-off and accommodating heel strike [20].

4. Classification

Some classification systems for calcaneus fractures have poor interobserver reliability, leading to difficulties in describing standardized treatment regimens [21]. Calcaneus fractures can be first classified based on whether they are extraarticular or intraarticular fractures, which account for approximately 25–40% and 60–75% of calcaneus fractures, respectively [22, 23]. Extraarticular calcaneus fractures are classified based on the location of the injury, including the anterior process, the sustentaculum tali, and the calcaneal tuberosity (which can be further classified with the Beavis classification).

The Beavis classification is based on the fracture morphology of the calcaneus tuberosity (**Figure 2**). A type 1 fracture or "Sleeve" fracture is an avulsion of the Achilles tendon with a small shell of cortical bone from the tuberosity. Type 2 or "Beak" fractures have oblique fracture lines that run posteriorly from the most superior portion of the posterior facet. Type 3 or "Infrabursal" fractures are avulsion fractures from the middle of the tuberosity.

Intra-articular calcaneus fractures can be classified with the Essex-Lopresti or the Sanders classification. The Essex-Lopresti classification is based on fracture lines using lateral radiograph images [24]. The primary fracture line runs through the posterior facet. The fracture is classified as tongue-type or depressed based on whether the secondary posteriorly exiting fracture line travels through or inferior to the calcaneal tubercle, respectively. However, the Essex-Lopresti classification has poor interobserver reliability [25].

The Sanders classification system uses coronal computed tomography (CT) scan images to determine the number of articular fragments at the widest point of the posterior facet at the level of the sustentaculum tali (**Figure 3**) [26, 27]. Sanders type I fractures are nondisplaced or have less than 2 mm of displacement, while type II fractures have one fracture line in the posterior facet with displacement. They are further separated into A, B, or C based on the primary fracture line location from lateral to medial. Type III fractures have two fracture lines in the posterior facet and are further separated into AB, AC, or BC based on the two fracture lines. Type IV fractures have three or more fracture lines.

The Crosby-Fitzgibbons system is another classification system based on CT imaging and was developed prior to the Sanders classification [10, 28]. The Crosby-Fitzgibbons classification system divides intra-articular facet fractures into three types. Nondisplaced or minimally displaced fractures are type I. More than 2 mm of

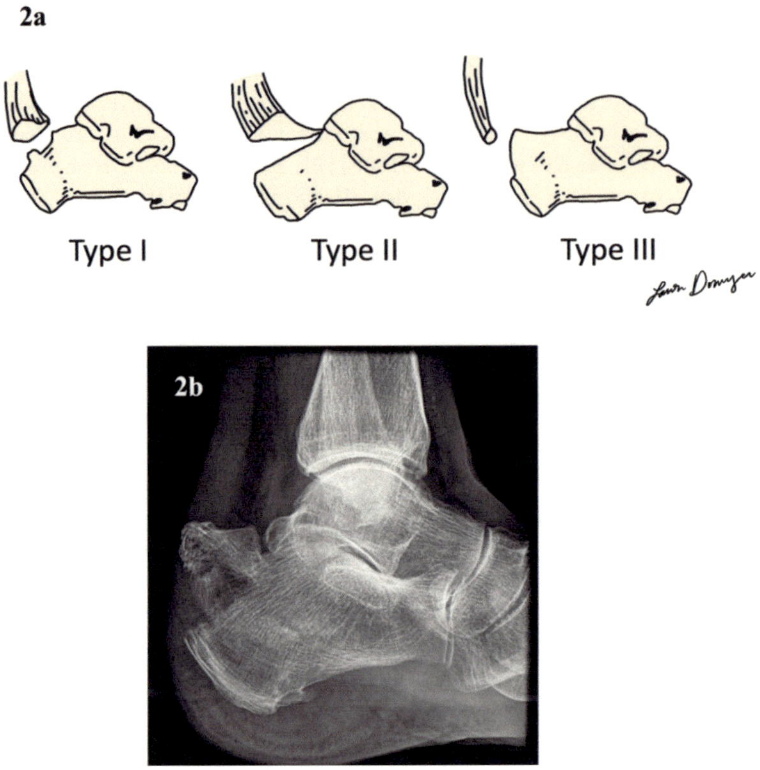

Figure 2.
Beavis classification. (a) Illustration of Beavis classification of extra-articular calcaneus fractures. (b) Radiographic example of a type 2 "beak" fracture.

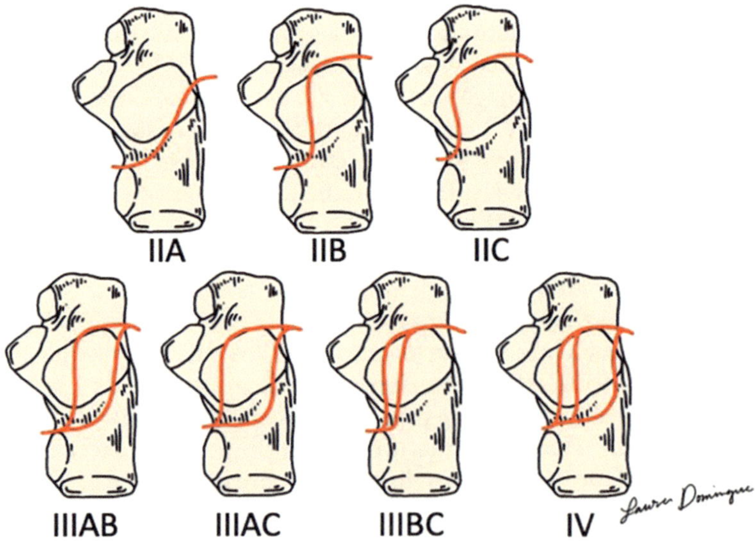

Figure 3.
Sanders classification of intra-articular calcaneus fractures.

displacement or subtalar joint depression are classified as type II and comminuted fractures as type III. Lauder et al. [28] compared the Sanders classification to the Crosby-Fitzgibbons system and found that the Crosby-Fitzgibbons system had significantly greater interobserver reliability than the Sanders classification. Swords et al. [29]. compared the Crosby-Fitzgibbons to the Eastwood and Sanders classifications and found no significant difference in the ability to predict patient functional

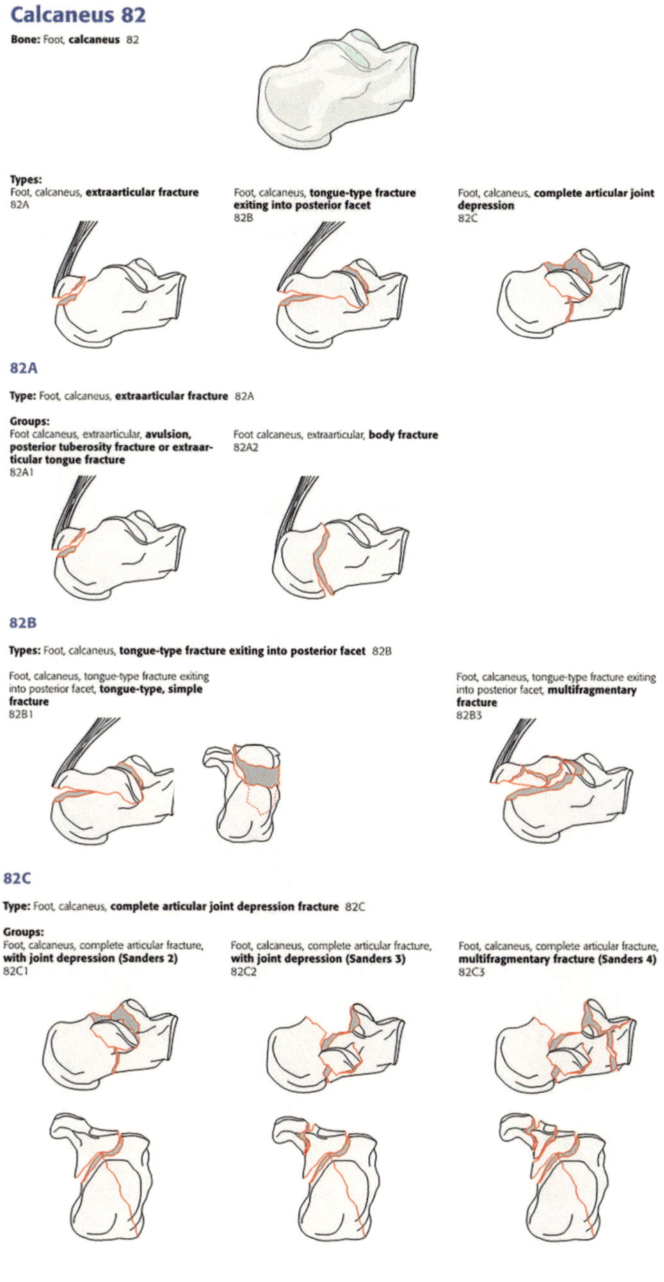

Figure 4.
AO/OTA fracture classification of calcaneus fractures [30].

outcomes using the Musculoskeletal Functional Assessment. However, the Sanders classification trended toward significance and had the highest predictive capability of functional outcomes.

The Müller/AO/OTA classification denotes the calcaneus as 82 and subdivides it into 82A, 82B, and 82C (**Figure 4**) [30]. Extraarticular fractures are classified as 82A, which is further divided into 82A1 for avulsion, posterior tuberosity, or extraarticular tongue-type fractures and 82A2 for extraarticular body fractures. Tongue-type fractures that exit into the posterior facet are classified as 82B1, 82B2 if there is associated joint depression, or 82B3 if highly comminuted. Complete articular fractures are classified as 82C. When there is joint depression with a single fracture line through the posterior facet, it is 82C1. If there is joint depression with two fracture lines (Sanders III equivalent), it is 82C2 and if highly comminuted (Sanders IV), 82C3.

The Regazzoni classification is a Swiss model for classifying calcaneal fractures [10, 31]. The Regazzoni classification system is based on coronal CT images. Type A fractures are peripheral fractures that are either extraarticular (A1), avulsion fractures of the sustentaculum (A2), or fractures of the anterior process (A3). Type B fractures are fractures involving the talocalcaneal joint. Type B fractures

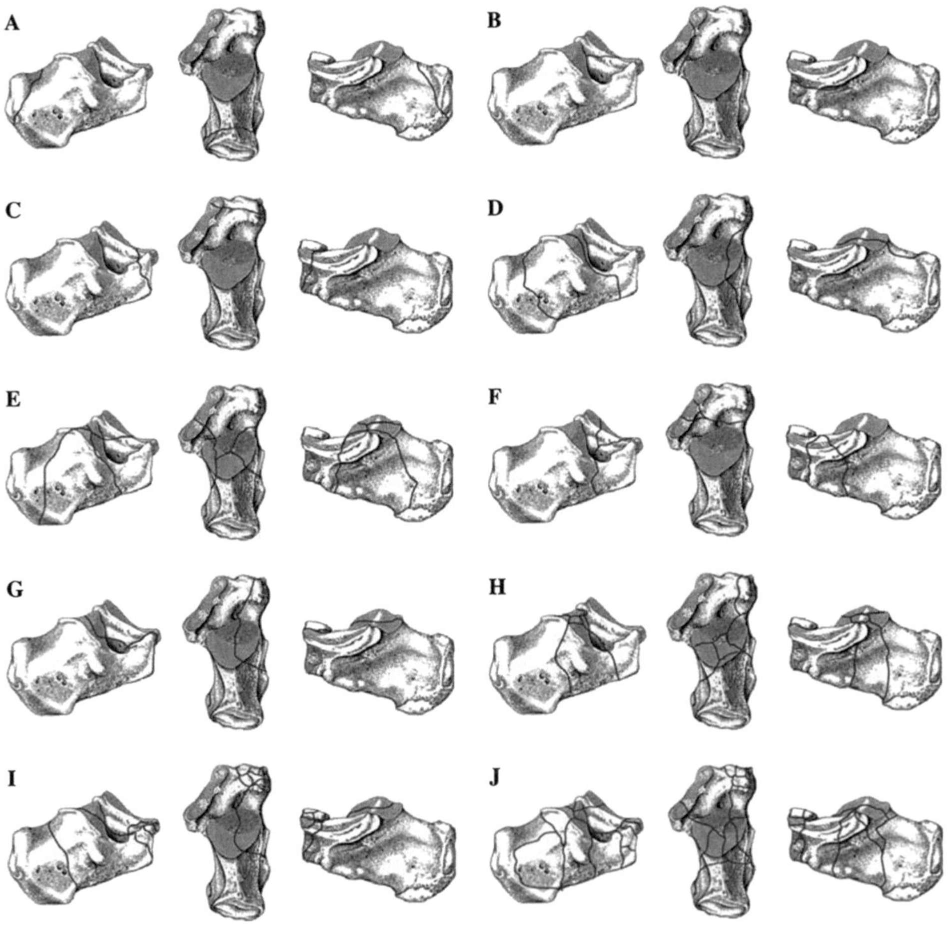

Figure 5.
Regazzoni classification of intra-articular calcaneal fractures [32].

can be those with single posterior facet fracture lines (B1), multiple posterior facet fractures (B2), and fractures involving the tarsal sinus (B3). Type C fractures are fractures of the talocalcaneal and calcaneocuboid joints. Single fracture lines in both joints constitute a C1 fracture. If one joint has multiple fracture lines or the tarsal sinus is involved, it is termed a C2 fracture. If multiple fracture lines involve both joints, it is a C3 fracture (**Figure 5**).

Rubino et al. [32]. compared the Essex-Lopresti, AO/OTA, Swiss Regazzoni, and Sanders classifications utilizing the American Orthopedic Foot and Ankle Society (AOFAS) hindfoot score, Creighton Nebraska Health Musculoskeletal Functional Assessment (MFA) Questionnaire, and other scores to determine the classification system with the best outcomes. Overall, the CT-based classifications had the highest prognostic values, particularly the Regazzoni and Sanders classifications.

5. Clinical evaluation/presentation

A thorough history and physical exam are essential for diagnosing calcaneus fractures. Important considerations of the patient's medical history, toxic habits, and daily activities (work status) are crucial as they affect outcomes. Pain and swelling are usually the first sign that a calcaneus fracture is present. Patients with these fractures may have other associated injuries that cause pain, which can lead to a delay in identifying calcaneus fractures. Although a rare occurrence in the authors' experiences, it has been reported that up to 10% of calcaneus fractures can lead to compartment syndrome [33]. Key components of the physical exam include visual inspection, neurovascular examination, and tendon function. Examination should include palpation and range of motion of the entire ipsilateral extremity and spine.

During visual inspection, ecchymosis and swelling of the heel, open skin lesions, or fracture blisters may be present. Tenting or ecchymosis may be visible in tuberosity fractures of the posterior calcaneus (**Figure 6**). Urgent surgical reduction is required if these findings are present to prevent posterior heel skin necrosis. Open skin lesions can present with calcaneus fractures (**Figure 7**). Urgent intravenous antibiotics, tetanus vaccination, and bedside irrigation are performed when open fracture is identified. After these urgent measures are taken, operative irrigation and debridement should be performed within 24 hours with concurrent temporary fixation with percutaneous pins, splinting, or definitive fixation with ORIF (described later in the chapter). Wound complications resulting from calcaneus fractures can be devastating and may require a free flap or amputation. Poor splinting techniques can contribute to posterior heel wounds. Therefore, to reduce the risk of splint/cast-related wounds, equinus can be allowed, and abundant heel padding is helpful.

Palpation typically elicits diffuse tenderness; in beak fractures, there will be a lack of posterior heel blanching. In avulsion fractures, there will be a heel cord continuity disruption. The neurovascular exam should include a comparison of the dorsalis pedis and posterior tibial pulses to the contralateral leg. Evidence of vascular insufficiency in the foot may require angiography or Doppler scanning. The primary targets when assessing tendon function should be the Achilles tendon and flexor hallucis longus (FHL). Decreased ankle plantarflexion strength occurs with avulsion of the posterior tuberosity, and weak flexion of the great toe points toward a displaced fracture entrapping the FHL.

Patients may also present with undiagnosed heel pain at times with negative radiographs. Concern for stress fractures should be present, especially in at-risk

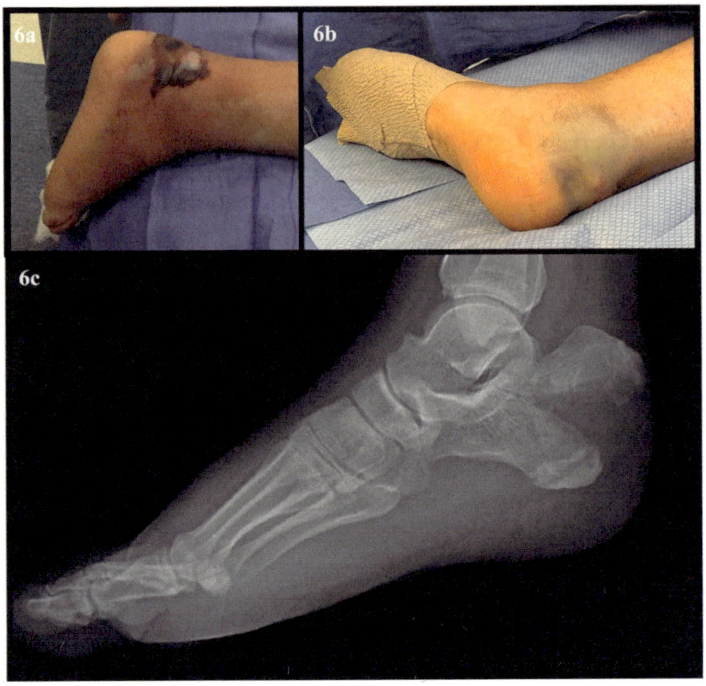

Figure 6.
Ecchymosis and fracture blisters due to tongue-type fracture. (a) Fracture blister and ecchymosis of the heel. (b) Ecchymosis of the heel due to a tongue-type fracture. (c) Radiograph of tongue-type fracture causing skin problems in (a).

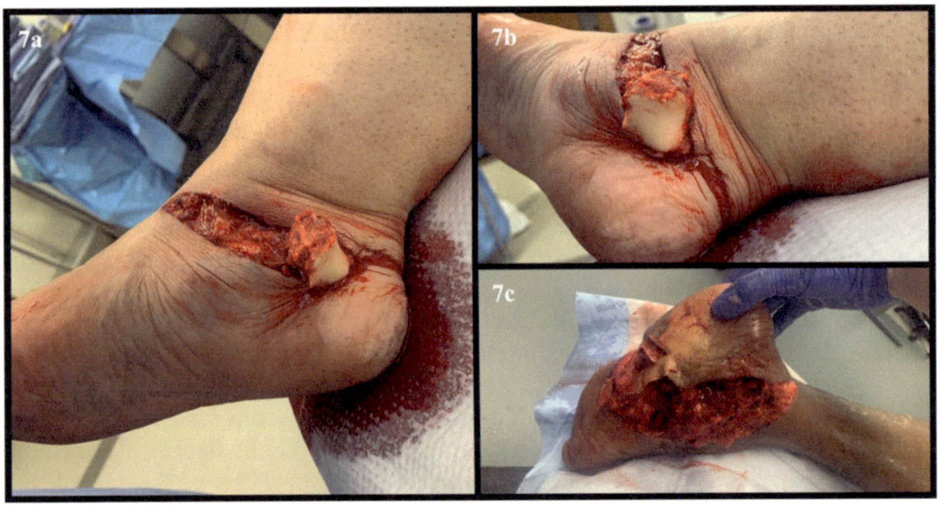

Figure 7.
Open calcaneal fractures. (a)-(c)-open skin lesions due to calcaneal fractures.

populations, including those with sudden increased physical activity, osteoporosis, or female athlete triad (menstrual dysfunction, low energy availability, and low bone mineral density).

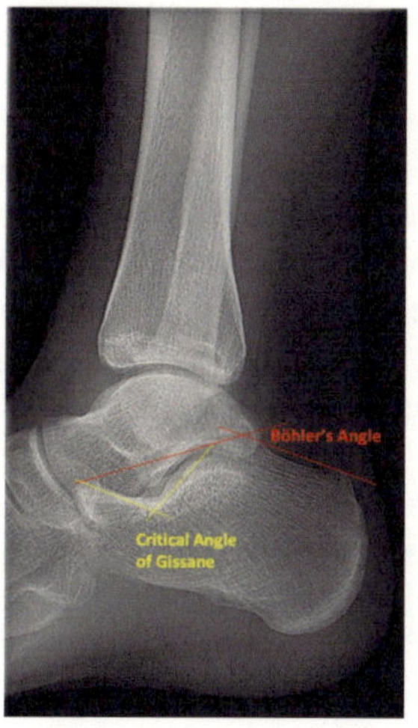

Figure 8.
Radiograph showing Böhler's angle and the critical angle of Gissane.

6. Radiographic evaluation

Standard ankle X-rays, including AP, lateral, and oblique views, can be supplemented with Harris and Broden views if there is a suspicion of a calcaneus fracture [34]. The Broden view visualizes the posterior calcaneus facet and subtalar joint, while the Harris view examines the tuberosity fragment, allowing for further characterization of the fracture. Radiographic measurements such as Böhler's angle and the Critical Angle of Gissane, normally between 20–40° and 120–145°, respectively, are important for identifying a collapse of the posterior facet (**Figure 8**). Still, normal measurements do not rule out a fracture.

CT scans are the gold standard for diagnosing calcaneus fractures and can guide surgical planning. CT scans are used to determine the Sanders classification as described above and provide additional detail regarding fragment size, displacement, and extent of intra-articular involvement beyond what is seen on plain radiographs. Magnetic resonance imaging (MRI) can be useful for calcaneus stress fractures. This should be considered when X-rays are normal, but there is high suspicion based on symptomatology, particularly in physically active patients [35, 36]. Furthermore, bone scintigraphy can be useful in individuals with metallic devices that would preclude MRI [37].

7. Treatment

Management of calcaneus fractures varies based on many factors. Nonoperative treatment is often recommended in extra-articular fractures with fragment size <1 cm in addition to less than 2 mm of displacement with an intact Achilles tendon. Nonoperative management is also indicated for Sanders Type I intra-articular fractures. Nonoperative management will typically consist of splinting and non-weight-bearing or toe-touch weight-bearing for 6–8 weeks with early range of motion of the ankle and hind foot to prevent stiffness [38, 39].

There is debate in the current literature on whether many calcaneus fractures are best managed with open reduction internal fixation (ORIF) or nonoperatively [10, 39–44]. ORIF has been shown to have greater rates of complications and repeat surgeries but with better outcomes regarding time to return to work and shoe fitting. ORIF was most beneficial in fracture patterns associated with fibular impingement, lateral comminution, and Böhler angles between 0° and 14° [40, 44]. Nonoperative management increases the risk of late subtalar fusion by 550–600% due to symptomatic subtalar arthritis [45, 46]. Additionally, without initial fixation and restoration of calcaneal height, the later subtalar fusion procedure increases in complexity due to the deformity created by the malunion of the calcaneus. The economic impact of treatment decisions must also be weighed. Concerning the impact on US healthcare payers, ORIF treatment costs almost $5000 less compared to nonoperative management over 5 years [47].

Operative management typically consists of ORIF, although external fixation for treatment of the calcaneus is well described (as discussed later in this chapter). ORIF can be performed through a traditional extensile lateral approach or minimally invasive approaches (**Figure 9**). Operative treatment aims to restore heel height and width, correct varus, and realign the subtalar joint. Operative indications include displaced tongue-type fractures with >1 cm of displacement; Sanders Type II, III, and IV fractures with articular displacement >1 mm; anterior process fracture with >25% involvement of calcaneocuboid joint; and displaced sustentaculum fractures [48].

Historically, ORIF has utilized the extensile lateral approach. This approach allows for excellent visualization of the subtalar joint by creating a full-thickness superior flap. It allows for the placement of a perimeter plate with fixation into the peripheral (more dense) bone of the entire calcaneus. The sural nerve and peroneal tendons are at risk during the approach and should be preserved. Meticulous and gentle soft-tissue handling should be observed (the so-called "no touch technique") [49].

Due to the risk of complications with ORIF, less invasive surgical techniques, such as percutaneous pinning, limited-incision sinus tarsi technique, and arthroscopic-assisted reduction and internal fixation, have been explored for fractures previously treated with the extensile lateral approach [50, 51]. While initially, the use of less invasive techniques had limited indications, these approaches have been shown to have equal clinical and radiographic outcomes to the extensile lateral approach with less wound-healing complications for all intra-articular calcaneal fractures [39, 51–53].

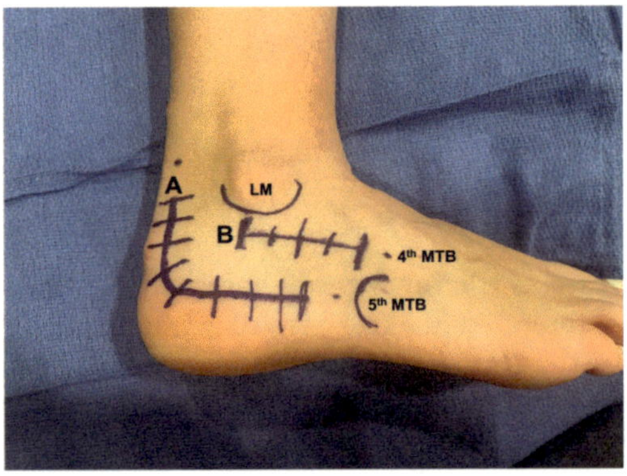

Figure 9.
Extensile lateral approach (A) and sinus tarsi (B) approaches to the calcaneus. MTB = Metatarsal Base, LM = lateral malleolus.

The sinus tarsi approach often utilizes a 2–4 cm incision over the sinus tarsi from 1 cm distal to the tip of the fibula toward the base of the fourth metatarsal. This approach provides direct visualization, reduction, and fixation of the posterior facet and calcaneocuboid joint while minimizing soft-tissue trauma [54]. This technique minimizes the risk of sural nerve injury and decreases surgical time and postoperative wound infections while enabling the surgeon visualization to restore the Böhler angle [51, 55–60]. The minimally invasive longitudinal approach (MILA) is an evolution of the sinus tarsi approach that takes the incision 1.5 cm distal to the lateral malleolus from the base of the fourth metatarsal to 1 cm anterior to the Achilles [54]. MILA has shown improved outcomes compared to the traditional sinus tarsi approach when using perimeter plates and compression screws [61], except in highly comminuted Sanders type IV fractures where the sinus tarsi approach was superior, most likely due to better visualization of the posterior facet [61].

Percutaneous fixation can be achieved with or without utilizing the limited sinus tarsi approach [53, 62, 63]. Percutaneous fixation can be performed using a variety of techniques to reduce fragments and maintain fixation with an external fixator or cannulated screws (**Figure 10**).

Arthroscopic-assisted reduction and internal fixation (ARIF) has shown excellent outcomes [64–66]. However, this technique may require increased setup, technical difficulty, and soft-tissue swelling, although disposable arthroscopy systems exist that may allow for similar visualization without the inconvenience of full arthroscopy setup [65]. When comparing less invasive techniques, there is no reported difference in radiographic restoration of Böhler's angle and clinical outcomes (AOFAS scores) [53].

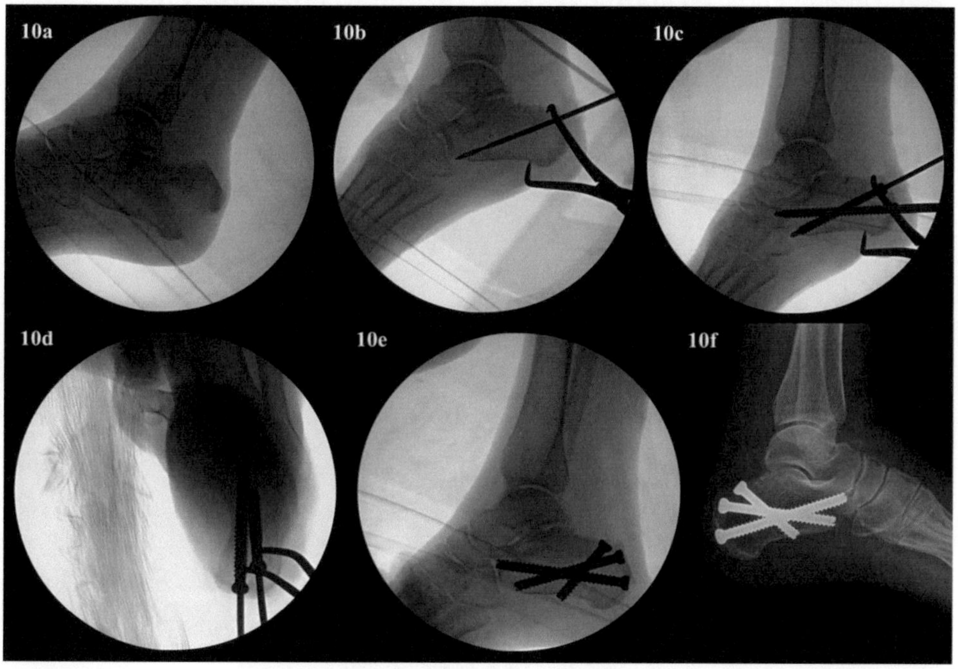

Figure 10.
Utilization of percutaneous pinning for the fixation of a tongue-type calcaneal fracture. (a) Displaced tongue-type calcaneal fracture. (b) Reduction of displaced tongue-type fracture using a Kirschner wire. (c) Partially threaded and fully threaded cannulated lag screw placement for fixation. (d) Harris view of cannulated screw placement. (e) Final operative radiographs. (f) Postoperative radiographs.

One study found an increased risk of secondary subtalar arthrodesis when performing percutaneous fixation due to subtalar osteoarthritis [67]. Percutaneous fixation is particularly indicated for patients with peripheral vascular disease or soft-tissue compromise in an attempt to avoid wound complications [52].

If these minimally invasive techniques are to be used, early treatment is indicated within 2 weeks due to early healing limiting fracture fragment mobility after this point [63]. Several studies have shown that minimally invasive approaches have decreased wound complications and secondary surgeries while having equivocal functional outcomes compared to ORIF [55, 57, 68].

In patients with severely comminuted Sanders type IV fractures, if ORIF alone is attempted, there is a high rate of clinically worse outcomes indicated by decreased AOFAS scores [69]. Sanders type IV fracture fixation can be done with ORIF alone, with some studies showing equal outcomes at 2-year follow-up when compared to ORIF with primary subtalar arthrodesis [69, 70]. However, beyond this time frame, there are decreased clinical outcomes utilizing the Short Form 36 version 2 (SF-36) scores requiring some patients with highly comminuted posterior facet calcaneus fractures treated with ORIF alone to undergo secondary subtalar arthrodesis [70]. Sanders et al. [43]. evaluated 10–20 year follow-up of ORIF treatment of Sanders type II and III fractures, showing a four times higher (18.6 vs. 47.4%) need for secondary subtalar fusion in type III fractures compared to that in type II fractures. Thus, some authors have suggested performing ORIF to restore height plus primary subtalar arthrodesis to avoid increased treatment costs and time off from work in fractures with higher degrees of comminution (**Figure 11**) [38]. However, it is difficult to predict which patients within this group of calcaneus fractures will develop chronic pain and eventually go on to arthrodesis, and this form of treatment can be a cause of its own downsides such as loss of motion and adjacent joint arthritis.

The importance of urgent reduction with percutaneous or open fixation of skin-threatening fractures cannot be overstated. Patients who sustain open fractures necessitating debridement and provisional stabilization and those with skin tenting, evolving wounds, or tongue-type/beak fractures should be initially splinted in

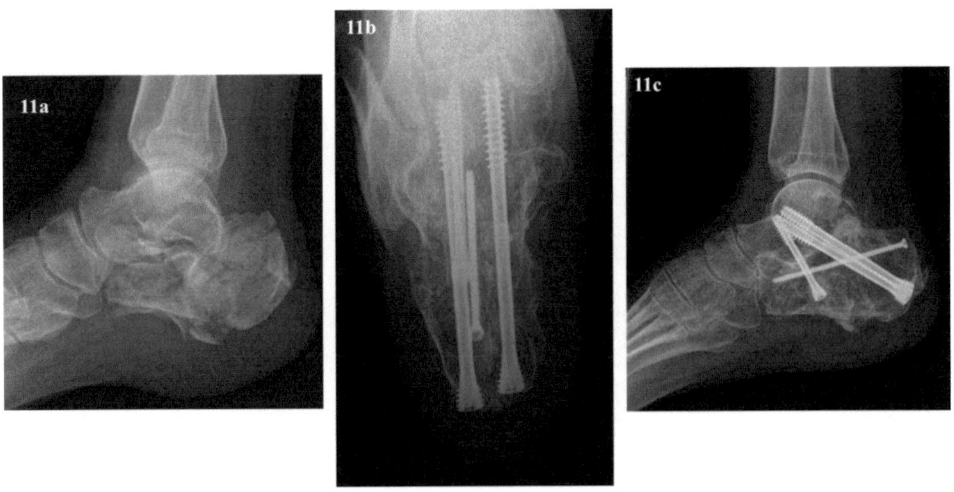

Figure 11.
Primary subtalar fusion. (a) Highly comminuted intra-articular calcaneal fracture. (b) Harris view of the calcaneus after primary subtalar fusion. (c) Lateral view of the calcaneus after primary subtalar fusion.

plantarflexion with abundant padding and then urgently addressed in the operating room in an attempt to prevent sequelae of skin necrosis and devastating wound complications.

External fixation is well described for calcaneus fractures in the literature as both a temporizing and definitive treatment option. With the high risk of soft-tissue complication with ORIF—even with minimally invasive approaches—external fixation has been further investigated as a treatment option. With the mechanism of action of calcaneus fractures primarily being due to high-energy trauma, the soft-tissue damage can be severe. Management often involves splinting the injury until the soft-tissue swelling has subsided. However, in more significantly displaced fractures, this delay in management can cause contraction of the soft tissues and preliminary callus formation [71–73]. These issues can combine to increase the overall difficulty of the surgical fixation for a calcaneus fracture [71–73]. As a result, there has been discussion in the literature of temporizing and definitive fixation of calcaneal fractures with external fixation.

Several external fixation methods have been proposed for calcaneal fractures, a testament to the lack of consensus and the overall difficulty of fracture management in these cases. Baumgaertel et al. described a minimally invasive external fixation approach of two-pin fixation, with one in each distal tibia and calcaneus to provide a distraction vector for the fracture, followed by lateral extensile ORIF [71]. The first pin is placed into the posterior calcaneus *via* a medial-to-lateral trajectory. The second pin is then placed either medial to lateral or anteriorly into the distal tibia. The pins are connected using an external fixator bar, and distraction force is applied. Overall alignment and reduction of the calcaneus is determined utilizing intraoperative X-ray and locked into position. The patients treated with external fixation followed by definitive fixation in their series had the external fixator in place for a median of 6.2 days [71]. The external fixator allowed for improved alignment and served as a reduction aid intraoperatively at the time of definitive fixation [71].

Githens et al. describe a medial-based fixator with pins in the proximal tibia, calcaneus, and midfoot to provide added construct stability while awaiting definitive fixation [73]. The first pin is placed across the midfoot medially, utilizing X-ray to ensure the tarsometatarsal joints are not violated with pin placement. The pin is placed across the medial, middle and into the body of the lateral cuneiform while under X-ray with a perfect AP view of the midfoot. The second pin is placed utilizing a medial to lateral trajectory into the distal tibia 1 cm above the incisura and parallel to the plafond. The third pin is placed into the calcaneus, typically the posterior tuberosity; however, the exact location of the pin can vary with fracture morphology. Importantly, the pin should be bicortical but not palpable on the lateral side. The first bar is placed between the tibia and the calcaneus, the second bar between the cuneiform and calcaneus, and the third between the tibia and cuneiforms (**Figure 12**) [73].

Ring frame external fixation combined with open operative approaches has been described in order to provide distraction, reduction of the articular surface, and internal fixation [74, 75]. Hou et al. describe the application of a ring frame external fixator utilizing 3, 2.5 mm Steinmann pins for fixation [75]. The first pin is placed transversely and perpendicular to the long axis of the tibia from lateral to medial at the junction of the middle and distal third of the tibia. The second pin is placed through the midfoot and the third through the posterior tuberosity of the calcaneus. The calcaneus and midfoot pins are each connected to separate half rings of the external fixator. The tibial pin is connected to a full ring of the external fixator. Connecting rods are placed between the tibial ring and the half rings of the midfoot and calcaneus. The midfoot

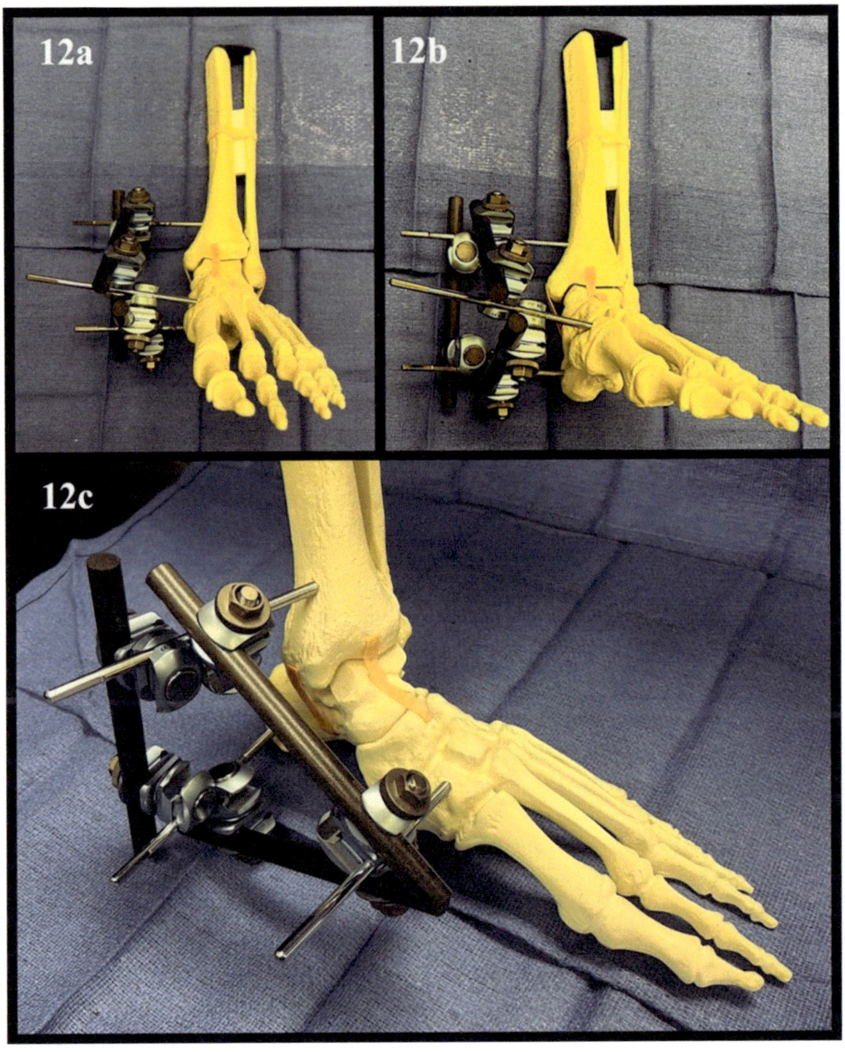

Figure 12.
Calcaneus fracture external fixation technique as described by Githens et al. [73]. (a)-(c) sawbones demonstration of the medial-based calcaneal external fixator setup.

and calcaneus half rings are joined *via* a single connecting rod directly inferior to the foot. Once the connecting rods are attached, they are left loose in order to perform the reduction. Utilizing intraoperative X-ray, the reduction is confirmed prior to locking the connecting rods. Once calcaneus length, height, Böhler's angle, and overall varus/valgus alignment are confirmed to be satisfactory, the limb is no longer manipulated and allowed to rest for 10 minutes. The goal of the 10-minute rest is to allow soft-tissue relaxation. After 10 minutes, an extensile lateral approach is utilized for fracture fixation. Once fixation is achieved, the external fixator is removed [75]. The senior author of the current chapter (JTR) has utilized a similar ring frame construct utilizing skinny wires, half pins, and external fixator struts in order to bring the calcaneus fracture out to length as temporary or definitive management (**Figure 13**).

Fu et al. described a series of patients treated with fixator-assisted reduction. Their patients were initially treated conservatively with rest, elevation, ice, and

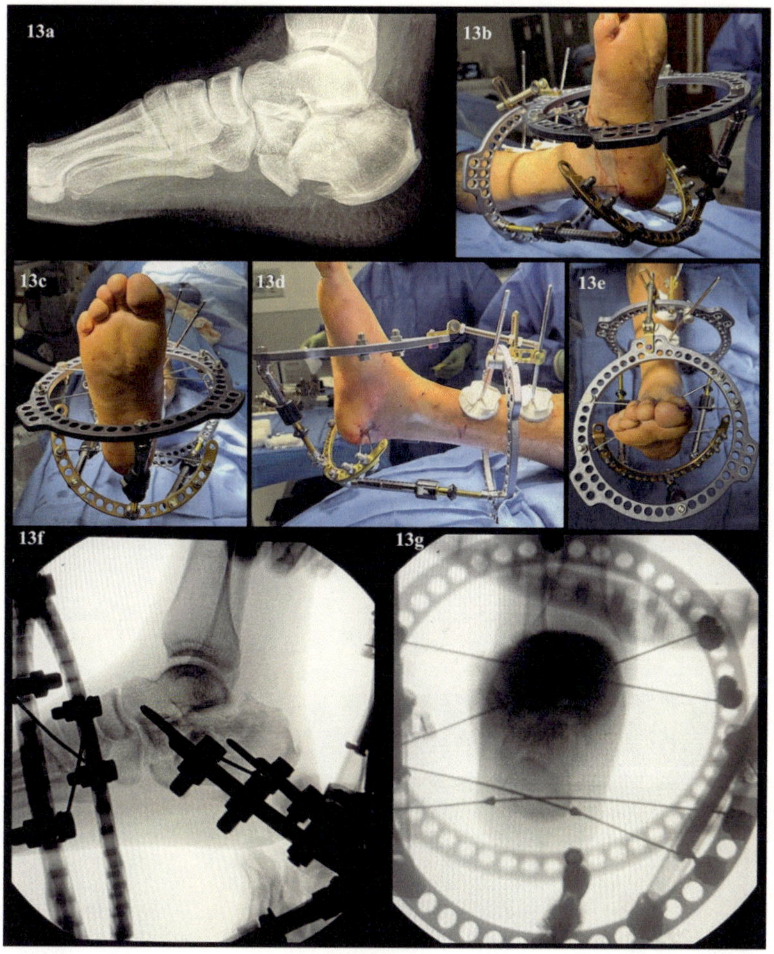

Figure 13.
Calcaneus ring frame technique (JTR). (a) Preoperative X-rays. (b–d) Clinical pictures of ring frame, skinny wires/tibial half pins, and struts. Wires are utilized for fixation into the calcaneal tuberosity and into the midfoot, while half pins provide tibial fixation. After rings have been connected to wires/pins, the calcaneus can be manipulated (pulled out to length and out of varus) and struts locked. (f–g) Postoperative external fixation X-rays.

compressive bandages with planned operative management to follow [74]. Splinting materials were not used, and ankle and foot motion was encouraged to reduce swelling. Once the swelling had subsided, operative treatment was performed. A lateral extensile approach was utilized, and an external fixator was applied to aid in reduction. With their technique, two transcalcaneal full pins are placed in the posterior calcaneus, with two half pins placed anterior-posterior into the distal tibia (**Figure 14**). Once adequate internal fixation is achieved, the external fixator is locked with the ankle in a neutral position. The external fixator remains in place for approximately 3 months postoperatively [74].

Studies have also discussed using external fixation as the definitive treatment of these fractures. Checa-Betagón et al. described a series of 38 patients where external fixation was utilized as the definitive treatment [76]. In their series, they utilize a lateral-based external fixator (OrthoFix™ Calcaneal Fixator) with six half pins (3 pin clusters) placed into the calcaneus (posterior tuberosity, subchondral bone of

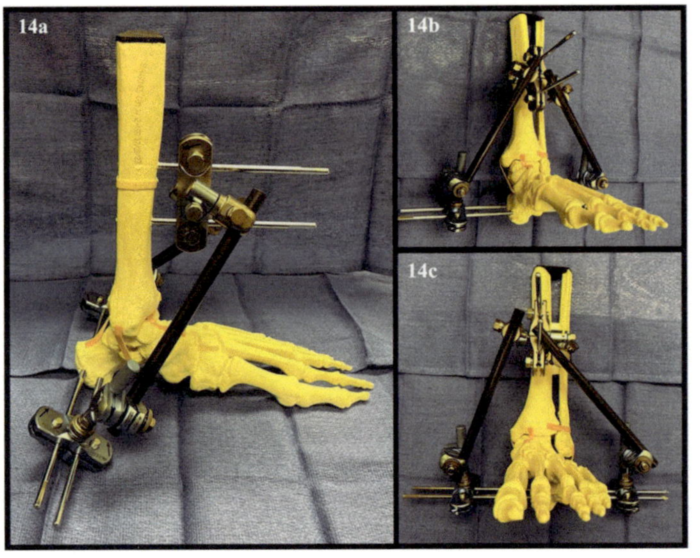

Figure 14.
Calcaneus fracture external fixation technique as described by Fu et al. [74]. (a)–(c) sawbones demonstration of external fixator setup for use in fixator-assisted delayed ORIF.

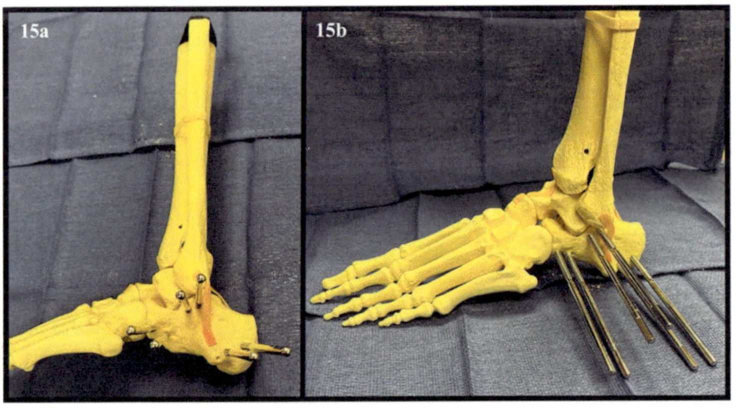

Figure 15.
Calcaneus fracture external fixation technique as described by Checa-Betagón et al. [76]. (a) and (b) sawbones demonstration of the pin sites for lateral-based OrthoFix™ external fixator for use in definitive treatment.

the posterior facet, or available subtalar surface) and the anterior tuberosity of the calcaneus or the cuboid (**Figure 15**). Pin clusters are placed in line with the X-ray beam when a perfect lateral view of each structure is seen individually. 69% of cases were reduced indirectly, while the remaining 31% required a minimal sinus tarsi approach or percutaneous k-wire joysticks to assist with reduction. They report results of external fixation to be similar to ORIF while reducing the risk of soft-tissue complication [76].

8. Treatment algorithm

The following treatment algorithm was created to aid in successfully managing calcaneus fractures (**Figure 16**).

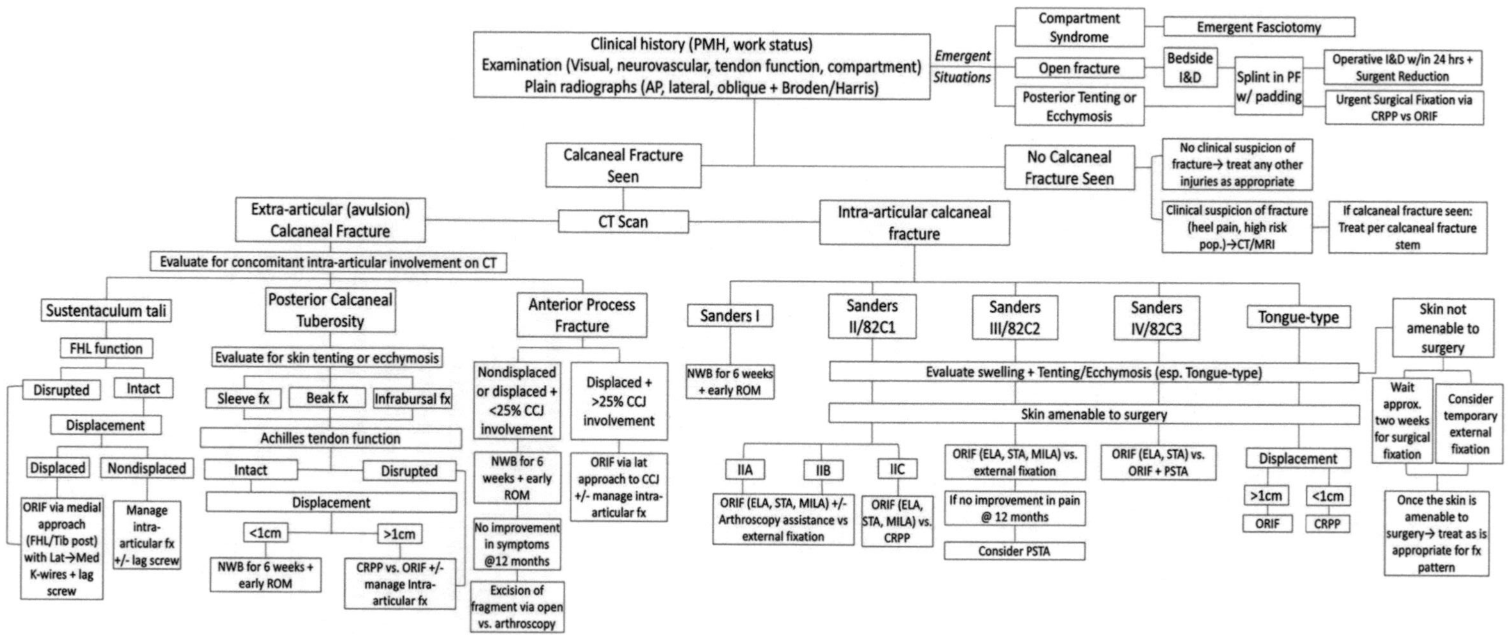

Figure 16.
Treatment algorithm for calcaneus fractures. (PF = plantarflexion, ORIF = operative reduction and internal fixation, PSTA = primary subtalar arthrodesis, NWB = non-weight-bearing, ROM = range of motion, ELA = extensile lateral approach, STA = sinus tarsi approach, MILA = minimally invasive longitudinal approach, FHL = flexor hallucis longus, FWB = full weight-bearing, CRPP = closed reduction and percutaneous pinning, CCJ = calcaneocuboid joint, fx = fracture.

9. Complications

Calcaneus fractures are prone to many complications based on the high-energy nature of these injuries and the calcaneus's thin, soft tissue envelope and anatomic relationship to many soft-tissue structures. Predominant complications consist of post-traumatic arthritis and wound-healing issues. Up to 37 and 20% of operations utilizing the extended L-shaped lateral incision have wound difficulties [50].

Long-term follow-up indicates that patients who undergo fixation of Sanders type III fractures are four times more likely to require subtalar arthrodesis compared to those with type II fractures [43]. This can be attributed to both the difficulty associated with treating these fractures and a testament to the overall high-energy mechanism responsible for most of these fractures. Inadequate articular reduction of the posterior facet can result in progressive loss of the joint [77]. Furthermore, subtalar arthritis can arise even with an anatomic articular reduction due to the chondrocyte damage sustained during the initial injury [77, 78]. Management of post-traumatic arthritis begins with conservative treatments similar to other joints. Over-the-counter anti-inflammatories, shoe-wear modification, bracing, activity modification, and other conservative modalities are first attempted. As conservative management fails, surgical options to be explored involve arthrodesis of the subtalar joint and other joints affected with post-traumatic arthritis.

Wound-healing problems represent one of the most common complications following surgical treatment of calcaneus fractures, with reports citing complication rates up to 25% [79–81]. The strongest risk factors for wound breakdown include diabetes, smoking, increasing Sanders type, and open fracture [79, 80]. Management of wound complications initially involves oral antibiotic therapy with local wound care for minor wounds. As the size of the wound increases beyond minor dehiscence, operative intervention is required, utilizing increasing levels of surgical debridement and soft-tissue reconstruction. Cavadas et al. propose an algorithm of soft-tissue management in calcaneal fractures utilizing a local subcutaneous transverse flap, a sural subcutaneous flap, and a distal vastus lateralis free flap, depending on the wound severity and patient factors [82]. The study defined minor wounds as <1.5 cm, moderate as 1.5–5 cm, and extensive as >5 cm. All wounds and fractures healed in the study [82]. Furthermore, Krishna et al. provide an algorithm for treating heel wounds utilizing wound location and weight-bearing status as a guide for soft-tissue reconstruction selection [83]. Local rotation and advancement flaps were very useful for small defects. Moderate anterior heel defects were treated with a medial plantar artery flap, and complete defects were treated with an extended reverse sural flap. The islanded reverse sural flap was utilized for posterior heel defects [83].

Additionally, neurologic injury is a common complication experienced in calcaneal fractures. When utilizing an extensile lateral approach, the most common injury involves the sural nerve, specifically the sensory cutaneous nerve [77, 84]. With a medial approach, the tibial nerve is at risk, with the calcaneal branch being most at risk [84, 85]. Management of this injury initially involves medications, including gabapentin, shoe inserts to accommodate the area of injury, and physical therapy [77, 84]. When there is failure of conservative management of the nerve injury, operative neurolysis and burying of the nerve into deeper tissue can be employed [77, 85, 86]. Regarding nonsurgical treatment of calcaneal fractures, posterior tibial nerve entrapment is the most common neurologic complication [77]. Treatment of this entrapment involves the treatment pathway of nerve compression with conservative management initiated first, followed by surgical decompression if necessary.

Malunion of calcaneal fractures is a well-documented complication. Consequences of malunion include but are not limited to: increased heel width, subfibular impingement, tibiotalar impingement, varus/valgus deformity at the hindfoot, peroneal tendon dysfunction, and subtalar arthrosis [77, 86, 87]. For isolated lateral impingement symptoms, lateral wall decompression can provide good results. However, more complex deformities require further operative planning and management [87].

Flexor hallucis longus pathology remains another complication worth noting. Damage to the FHL tendon can occur due to displaced fracture and misplaced screws into the sustentaculum tali during reconstruction. Misplaced screws can penetrate the opposite cortex inferior at the sustentaculum tali and directly impinge on the FHL tendon [88]. Treatment involves screw removal and replacement in this setting.

10. Conclusion

Calcaneus fractures are common lower extremity fractures requiring a comprehensive knowledge of anatomy, an attentive clinical and radiographic evaluation, and an understanding of surgical techniques for appropriate management. Initial evaluation of calcaneus fractures must consider the mechanism of injury and the potential for associated injuries. As operative indications and treatment for calcaneus fractures continue to evolve, there is a focus on minimizing, delaying, or preventing arthritis while minimizing wound complications. External fixation can restore length, rotation, and alignment while decreasing the risks associated with internal fixation of calcaneus fractures. Sinus tarsi approaches also show promise with decreased soft-tissue complications and similar patient-reported outcomes. Wound breakdown remains the most significant and potentially devastating complication of these fractures. After wound complications, neurologic injury and other soft-tissue injuries are common, while malunion and its sequela are well-documented bony complications.

Acknowledgements

The authors would like to thank Lauren Domingue, for the drawings of the Anatomic Landmarks of the Calcaneus, Beavis fracture classification, and Sanders fracture classification. The authors would like to thank Mark Hetzer and Isabelle Annaheim from Synthes GmbH, Oberdorf, Switzerland, for the drawings of the Regazzoni [31] fracture classification. The authors would also like to thank Synthes for providing the external fixator equipment and sawbones used in demonstrations.

Author details

McKenna W. Box[1], Grayson A. Domingue[2], Neil J. Werthmann[3], Jan P. Szatkowski[4] and John T. Riehl[3]*

1 University of Oklahoma College of Medicine, USA

2 Department of Orthopaedic Surgery, University of Oklahoma Health Sciences Center, Oklahoma City, Oklahoma, USA

3 Department of Orthopaedic Surgery, Medical City UNT/TCU Orthopaedic Surgery Residency Program, USA

4 Department of Orthopaedic Surgery, Indiana University Health, USA

*Address all correspondence to: jtriehl@hotmail.com

References

[1] Eiff MP, Hatch RL. Fracture Management for Primary Care and Emergency Medicine. 4th ed. Amsterdam: Elsevier; 2020

[2] Italiano J, Bitterman AD. Diagnosis and management of calcaneal stress fractures. Radiologic Technology. 2021;**93**(2):177-194

[3] Zhu Y, Li J, Liu S, et al. Socioeconomic factors and lifestyles influencing the incidence of calcaneal fractures, a national population-based survey in China. Journal of Orthopaedic Surgery and Research. 2019;**14**(1):423. DOI: 10.1186/s13018-019-1493-2

[4] Mitchell MJ, McKinley JC, Robinson CM. The epidemiology of calcaneal fractures. Foot (Edinburgh, Scotland). 2009;**19**(4):197-200. DOI: 10.1016/j.foot.2009.05.001

[5] Herrera-Pérez M, Oller-Boix A, Valderrabano V, et al. Calcaneal fractures: Controversies and consensus. Acta Ortopédica Mexicana. 2018;**32**(3):172-181 Fracturas de calcáneo: controversias y consensos

[6] Lowery RB, Calhoun JH. Fractures of the calcaneus. Part I: Anatomy, injury mechanism, and classification. Foot & Ankle International. 1996;**17**(4):230-235. DOI: 10.1177/107110079601700409

[7] Bohl DD, Ondeck NT, Samuel AM, et al. Demographics, mechanisms of injury, and concurrent injuries associated with calcaneus fractures: A study of 14 516 patients in the American College of Surgeons National Trauma Data Bank. Foot & Ankle Specialist. 2017;**10**(5):402-410. DOI: 10.1177/1938640016679703

[8] Hall RL, Shereff MJ. Anatomy of the calcaneus. Clinical Orthopaedics and Related Research. 1993;**290**:27-35

[9] Keener BJ, Sizensky JA. The anatomy of the calcaneus and surrounding structures. Foot and Ankle Clinics. 2005;**10**(3):413-424. DOI: 10.1016/j.fcl.2005.04.003

[10] Agren PH, Wretenberg P, Sayed-Noor AS. Operative versus nonoperative treatment of displaced intra-articular calcaneal fractures: A prospective, randomized, controlled multicenter trial. The Journal of Bone and Joint Surgery. American Volume. 2013;**95**(15):1351-1357. DOI: 10.2106/jbjs.L.00759

[11] Viladot A, Lorenzo JC, Salazar J, Rodríguez A. The subtalar joint: Embryology and morphology. Foot & Ankle. 1984;**5**(2):54-66. DOI: 10.1177/107110078400500203

[12] Klein MA, Spreitzer AM. MR imaging of the tarsal sinus and canal: Normal anatomy, pathologic findings, and features of the sinus tarsi syndrome. Radiology. 1993;**186**(1):233-240. DOI: 10.1148/radiology.186.1.8416571

[13] Al-Ashhab ME, Elgazzar AS. Treatment for displaced sustentaculum tali fractures. Foot (Edinburgh, Scotland). 2018;**35**:70-74. DOI: 10.1016/j.foot.2017.12.002

[14] Della Rocca GJ, Nork SE, Barei DP, Taitsman LA, Benirschke SK. Fractures of the sustentaculum tali: Injury characteristics and surgical technique for reduction. Foot & Ankle International. 2009;**30**(11):1037-1041. DOI: 10.3113/fai.2009.1037

[15] Dürr C, Zwipp H, Rammelt S. Fractures of the sustentaculum tali. Operative Orthopädie und Traumatologie. 2013;**25**(6):569-578. DOI: 10.1007/s00064-013-0247-2

[16] Gitajn IL, Abousayed M, Toussaint RJ, Ting B, Jin J, Kwon JY. Anatomic alignment and integrity of the Sustentaculum Tali in intra-articular calcaneal fractures: Is the Sustentaculum Tali truly constant? The Journal of Bone and Joint Surgery. American Volume. 2014;**96**(12):1000-1005. DOI: 10.2106/jbjs.M.00330

[17] Gupton MÖM, Terreberry RR. Anatomy, Bony Pelvis and Lower Limb: Calcaneus. St. Petersburg, FL, USA: StatPearls Publishing; 2023. Available from: https://www.ncbi.nlm.nih.gov/books/NBK519544/ [Accessed: September 2, 2023]

[18] Donatelli RA. Normal biomechanics of the foot and ankle. The Journal of Orthopaedic and Sports Physical Therapy. 1985;**7**(3):91-95. DOI: 10.2519/jospt.1985.7.3.91

[19] Bolgla LA, Malone TR. Plantar fasciitis and the windlass mechanism: A biomechanical link to clinical practice. Journal of Athletic Training. 2004;**39**(1):77-82

[20] Koo S, Lee KM, Cha YJ. Plantar-flexion of the ankle joint complex in terminal stance is initiated by subtalar plantar-flexion: A bi-planar fluoroscopy study. Gait & Posture. 2015;**42**(4):424-429. DOI: 10.1016/j.gaitpost.2015.07.009

[21] Sanders R. Current concepts review - displaced intra-articular fractures of the calcaneus. JBJS. 2000;**82**(2):225-250

[22] Jiménez-Almonte JH, King JD, Luo TD, Aneja A, Moghadamian E. Classifications in brief: Sanders classification of intraarticular fractures of the calcaneus. Clinical Orthopaedics and Related Research. 2019;**477**(2):467-471. DOI: 10.1097/corr.0000000000000539

[23] Schepers T, Ginai AZ, Van Lieshout EM, Patka P. Demographics of extra-articular calcaneal fractures: Including a review of the literature on treatment and outcome. Archives of Orthopaedic and Trauma Surgery. 2008;**128**(10):1099-1106. DOI: 10.1007/s00402-007-0517-2

[24] Essex-Lopresti P. The mechanism, reduction technique, and results in fractures of the oscalcis. The British Journal of Surgery. 1952;**39**(157):395-419. DOI: 10.1002/bjs.18003915704

[25] Schepers T, van Lieshout EM, Ginai AZ, Mulder PG, Heetveld MJ, Patka P. Calcaneal fracture classification: A comparative study. The Journal of Foot and Ankle Surgery. 2009;**48**(2):156-162. DOI: 10.1053/j.jfas.2008.11.006

[26] Galluzzo M, Greco F, Pietragalla M, et al. Calcaneal fractures: Radiological and CT evaluation and classification systems. Acta Bio-Medica. 2018;**89**(1-s):138-150. DOI: 10.23750/abm.v89i1-S.7017

[27] Sanders R, Fortin P, DiPasquale T, Walling A. Operative treatment in 120 displaced intraarticular calcaneal fractures. Results using a prognostic computed tomography scan classification. Clinical Orthopaedics and Related Research. 1993;**290**:87-95

[28] Lauder AJ, Inda DJ, Bott AM, Clare MP, Fitzgibbons TC, Mormino MA. Interobserver and intraobserver reliability of two classification systems for intra-articular calcaneal fractures. Foot & Ankle International. 2006;**27**(4):251-255. DOI: 10.1177/107110070602700405

[29] Swords MP, Alton TB, Holt S, Sangeorzan BJ, Shank JR, Benirschke SK. Prognostic value of computed tomography classification systems for intra-articular calcaneus fractures. Foot & Ankle International. 2014;**35**(10):975-980. DOI: 10.1177/1071100714548196

[30] Marsh JL, Slongo TF, Agel J, et al. Fracture and dislocation classification compendium - 2007: Orthopaedic trauma association classification, database and outcomes committee. Journal of Orthopaedic Trauma. 2007;**21**(10 Suppl.):S1-S133. DOI: 10.1097/00005131-200711101-00001

[31] Regazzoni P. Behandlung von Kalkaneusfrakturen. Basler Beiträge Chir. 1991;**3**:49-62

[32] Rubino R, Valderrabano V, Sutter PM, Regazzoni P. Prognostic value of four classifications of calcaneal fractures. Foot & Ankle International. 2009;**30**(3):229-238. DOI: 10.3113/fai.2009.0229

[33] Myerson M, Manoli A. Compartment syndromes of the foot after calcaneal fractures. Clinical Orthopaedics and Related Research. 1993;**290**:142-150

[34] Buckley RE, Tough S. Displaced intra-articular calcaneal fractures. The Journal of the American Academy of Orthopaedic Surgeons. 2004;**12**(3):172-178. DOI: 10.5435/00124635-200405000-00005

[35] Niva MH, Sormaala MJ, Kiuru MJ, Haataja R, Ahovuo JA, Pihlajamaki HK. Bone stress injuries of the ankle and foot: An 86-month magnetic resonance imaging-based study of physically active young adults. The American Journal of Sports Medicine. 2007;**35**(4):643-649. DOI: 10.1177/0363546506295701

[36] Sormaala MJ, Niva MH, Kiuru MJ, Mattila VM, Pihlajamäki HK. Stress injuries of the calcaneus detected with magnetic resonance imaging in military recruits. The Journal of Bone and Joint Surgery. American Volume. 2006;**88**(10):2237-2242. DOI: 10.2106/jbjs.E.01447

[37] Ozdemir H, Ozdemir A, Söyücü Y, Urgüden M. The role of bone scintigraphy in determining the etiology of heel pain. Annals of Nuclear Medicine. 2002;**16**(6):395-401. DOI: 10.1007/bf02990077

[38] Sharr PJ, Mangupli MM, Winson IG, Buckley RE. Current management options for displaced intra-articular calcaneal fractures: Non-operative, ORIF, minimally invasive reduction and fixation or primary ORIF and subtalar arthrodesis. A contemporary review. Foot and Ankle Surgery. 2016;**22**(1):1-8. DOI: 10.1016/j.fas.2015.10.003

[39] Wei N, Yuwen P, Liu W, et al. Operative versus nonoperative treatment of displaced intra-articular calcaneal fractures: A meta-analysis of current evidence base. Medicine (Baltimore). 2017;**96**(49):e9027. DOI: 10.1097/md.0000000000009027

[40] Buckley R, Tough S, McCormack R, et al. Operative compared with nonoperative treatment of displaced intra-articular calcaneal fractures: A prospective, randomized, controlled multicenter trial. The Journal of Bone and Joint Surgery. American Volume. 2002;**84**(10):1733-1744. DOI: 10.2106/00004623-200210000-00001

[41] Dickenson EJ, Parsons N, Griffin DR. Open reduction and internal fixation versus nonoperative treatment for closed, displaced, intra-articular fractures of the calcaneus: Long-term follow-up from the HeFT randomized controlled trial. Bone Joint Journal. 2021;**103-b**(6):1040-1046. DOI: 10.1302/0301-620x.103b6.Bjj-2020-1962.R2

[42] Griffin D, Parsons N, Shaw E, et al. Operative versus non-operative treatment for closed, displaced, intra-articular fractures of the calcaneus:

Randomised controlled trial. BMJ. 2014;**349**:g4483. DOI: 10.1136/bmj.g4483

[43] Sanders R, Vaupel ZM, Erdogan M, Downes K. Operative treatment of displaced intraarticular calcaneal fractures: Long-term (10-20 years) results in 108 fractures using a prognostic CT classification. Journal of Orthopaedic Trauma. 2014;**28**(10):551-563. DOI: 10.1097/bot.0000000000000169

[44] Selim A, Ponugoti N, Chandrashekar S. Systematic review of operative vs nonoperative treatment of displaced Intraarticular calcaneal fractures. Foot & Ankle Orthopaedics. 2022;**7**(2):24730114221101609. DOI: 10.1177/24730114221101609

[45] Csizy M, Buckley R, Tough S, et al. Displaced intra-articular calcaneal fractures: Variables predicting late subtalar fusion. Journal of Orthopaedic Trauma. 2003;**17**(2):106-112. DOI: 10.1097/00005131-200302000-00005

[46] Radnay CS, Clare MP, Sanders RW. Subtalar fusion after displaced intra-articular calcaneal fractures: Does initial operative treatment matter? The Journal of Bone and Joint Surgery. American Volume. 2009;**91**(3):541-546. DOI: 10.2106/jbjs.G.01445

[47] Albin SR, Bellows BK, Van Boerum DH, et al. Cost-effectiveness of operative versus nonoperative Management of Patients with Intra-articular Calcaneal Fractures. Journal of Orthopaedic Trauma. 2020;**34**(7):382-388. DOI: 10.1097/bot.0000000000001731

[48] Allegra PR, Rivera S, Desai SS, Aiyer A, Kaplan J, Gross CE. Intra-articular calcaneus fractures: Current concepts review. Foot & Ankle Orthopaedics. 2020;**5**(3):2473011420927334. DOI: 10.1177/2473011420927334

[49] Schweitzer KM Jr, Gaskill TR, Easley ME, Nunley JA 2nd. Open reduction and internal fixation of intra-articular calcaneal fractures via an extensile lateral approach. Journal of Bone & Joint Surgery Essential Surgical Techniques. 2011;**1**(2):e7. DOI: 10.2106/jbjs.St.K.00012

[50] Hsu AR, Anderson RB, Cohen BE. Advances in surgical management of intra-articular calcaneus fractures. The Journal of the American Academy of Orthopaedic Surgeons. 2015;**23**(7):399-407. DOI: 10.5435/jaaos-d-14-00287

[51] Seat A, Seat C. Lateral extensile approach versus minimal incision approach for open reduction and internal fixation of displaced intra-articular calcaneal fractures: A meta-analysis. The Journal of Foot and Ankle Surgery. 2020;**59**(2):356-366. DOI: 10.1053/j.jfas.2019.08.007

[52] DeWall M, Henderson CE, McKinley TO, Phelps T, Dolan L, Marsh JL. Percutaneous reduction and fixation of displaced intra-articular calcaneus fractures. Journal of Orthopaedic Trauma. 2010;**24**(8):466-472. DOI: 10.1097/BOT.0b013e3181defd74

[53] Wallin KJ, Cozzetto D, Russell L, Hallare DA, Lee DK. Evidence-based rationale for percutaneous fixation technique of displaced intra-articular calcaneal fractures: A systematic review of clinical outcomes. The Journal of Foot and Ankle Surgery. 2014;**53**(6):740-743. DOI: 10.1053/j.jfas.2014.03.018

[54] Zhan J, Hu C, Zhu N, Fang W, Jing J, Wang G. A modified tarsal sinus approach for intra-articular calcaneal fractures. Journal of Orthopaedic Surgery (Hong Kong).

2019;**27**(2):2309499019836165. DOI: 10.1177/2309499019836165

[55] Jin C, Weng D, Yang W, He W, Liang W, Qian Y. Minimally invasive percutaneous osteosynthesis versus ORIF for Sanders type II and III calcaneal fractures: A prospective, randomized intervention trial. Journal of Orthopaedic Surgery and Research. 2017;**12**(1):10. DOI: 10.1186/s13018-017-0511-5

[56] Kikuchi C, Charlton TP, Thordarson DB. Limited sinus tarsi approach for intra-articular calcaneus fractures. Foot & Ankle International. 2013;**34**(12):1689-1694. DOI: 10.1177/1071100713510267

[57] Mehta CR, An VVG, Phan K, Sivakumar B, Kanawati AJ, Suthersan M. Extensile lateral versus sinus tarsi approach for displaced, intra-articular calcaneal fractures: A meta-analysis. Journal of Orthopaedic Surgery and Research. 2018;**13**(1):243. DOI: 10.1186/s13018-018-0943-6

[58] Nosewicz T, Knupp M, Barg A, et al. Mini-open sinus tarsi approach with percutaneous screw fixation of displaced calcaneal fractures: A prospective computed tomography-based study. Foot & Ankle International. 2012;**33**(11):925-933. DOI: 10.3113/fai.2012.0925

[59] Weber M, Lehmann O, Sägesser D, Krause F. Limited open reduction and internal fixation of displaced intra-articular fractures of the calcaneum. Journal of Bone and Joint Surgery. British Volume (London). 2008;**90**(12):1608-1616. DOI: 10.1302/0301-620x.90b12.20638

[60] Xia S, Lu Y, Wang H, Wu Z, Wang Z. Open reduction and internal fixation with conventional plate via L-shaped lateral approach versus internal fixation with percutaneous plate via a sinus tarsi approach for calcaneal fractures - A randomized controlled trial. International Journal of Surgery. 2014;**12**(5):475-480. DOI: 10.1016/j.ijsu.2014.03.001

[61] Zhang T, Su Y, Chen W, Zhang Q, Wu Z, Zhang Y. Displaced intra-articular calcaneal fractures treated in a minimally invasive fashion: Longitudinal approach versus sinus tarsi approach. The Journal of Bone and Joint Surgery. American Volume. 2014;**96**(4):302-309. DOI: 10.2106/jbjs.L.01215

[62] Ebraheim NA, Elgafy H, Sabry FF, Freih M, Abou-Chakra IS. Sinus tarsi approach with trans-articular fixation for displaced intra-articular fractures of the calcaneus. Foot & Ankle International. 2000;**21**(2):105-113. DOI: 10.1177/107110070002100203

[63] Stulik J, Stehlik J, Rysavy M, Wozniak A. Minimally-invasive treatment of intra-articular fractures of the calcaneum. Journal of Bone and Joint Surgery. British Volume (London). 2006;**88**(12):1634-1641. DOI: 10.1302/0301-620x.88b12.17379

[64] Gavlik JM, Rammelt S, Zwipp H. The use of subtalar arthroscopy in open reduction and internal fixation of intra-articular calcaneal fractures. Injury. 2002;**33**(1):63-71. DOI: 10.1016/s0020-1383(01)00077-8

[65] Sivakumar BS, Wong P, Dick CG, Steer RA, Tetsworth K. Arthroscopic reduction and percutaneous fixation of selected calcaneus fractures: Surgical technique and early results. Journal of Orthopaedic Trauma. 2014;**28**(10):569-576. DOI: 10.1097/bot.0000000000000157

[66] Woon CY, Chong KW, Yeo W, Eng-Meng Yeo N, Wong MK. Subtalar arthroscopy and flurosocopy in

percutaneous fixation of intra-articular calcaneal fractures: The best of both worlds. The Journal of Trauma. 2011;**71**(4):917-925. DOI: 10.1097/TA.0b013e318202f1d0

[67] Schepers T, Vogels LM, Schipper IB, Patka P. Percutaneous reduction and fixation of intraarticular calcaneal fractures. Operative Orthopädie und Traumatologie. 2008;**20**(2):168-175. DOI: 10.1007/s00064-008-1239-5

[68] Kline AJ, Anderson RB, Davis WH, Jones CP, Cohen BE. Minimally invasive technique versus an extensile lateral approach for intra-articular calcaneal fractures. Foot & Ankle International. 2013;**34**(6):773-780. DOI: 10.1177/1071100713477607

[69] Almeida JF, Vale C, Gonzalez T, Gomes TM, Oliva XM. Osteosynthesis or primary arthrodesis for displaced intra-articular calcaneus fractures Sanders type IV - A systematic review. Foot and Ankle Surgery. 2022;**28**(3):281-287. DOI: 10.1016/j.fas.2021.04.006

[70] Buckley R, Leighton R, Sanders D, et al. Open reduction and internal fixation compared with ORIF and primary subtalar arthrodesis for treatment of Sanders type IV calcaneal fractures: A randomized multicenter trial. Journal of Orthopaedic Trauma. 2014;**28**(10):577-583. DOI: 10.1097/bot.0000000000000191

[71] Baumgaertel FR, Gotzen L. Two-stage operative treatment of comminuted os calcis fractures. Primary indirect reduction with medial external fixation and delayed lateral plate fixation. Clinical Orthopaedics and Related Research. 1993;**290**:132-141

[72] Farrell BM, Lin CA, Moon CN. Temporising external fixation of calcaneus fractures prior to definitive plate fixation: A case series. Injury. 2015;**46**(Suppl. 3):S19-S22. DOI: 10.1016/s0020-1383(15)30006-1

[73] Githens M, Shatsky J, Agel J, Bransford RJ, Benirschke SK. Medial external fixation for staged treatment of closed calcaneus fractures: Surgical technique and case series. Journal of Orthopaedic Surgery (Hong Kong). 2017;**25**(3):2309499017727915. DOI: 10.1177/2309499017727915

[74] Fu TH, Liu HC, Su YS, Wang CJ. Treatment of displaced intra-articular calcaneal fractures with combined transarticular external fixation and minimal internal fixation. Foot & Ankle International. 2013;**34**(1):91-98. DOI: 10.1177/1071100712460364

[75] Hou J, Zhang N, Chen G, et al. Circular external fixator assisted open reduction combined with locking plate fixation for intra-articular Comminuted fractures of the calcaneus. The Journal of Foot and Ankle Surgery. 2023;**62**(3):437-443. DOI: 10.1053/j.jfas.2022.10.009

[76] Checa-Betegón P, Valle-Cruz J, Llanos-Sanz S, Miguel-Miguel C, Sánchez-Del-Saz J, García-Coiradas J. External fixation in intra-articular fractures of the calcaneus: Is it a valid option as definitive treatment? European Journal of Orthopaedic Surgery and Traumatology. Jan 2024;**34**(1):201-208. DOI: 10.1007/s00590-023-03621-y

[77] Clare MP, Crawford WS. Managing complications of calcaneus fractures. Foot and Ankle Clinics. 2017;**22**(1):105-116. DOI: 10.1016/j.fcl.2016.09.007

[78] Sanders R. Intra-articular fractures of the calcaneus: Present state of the art. Journal of Orthopaedic Trauma. 1992;**6**(2):252-265. DOI: 10.1097/00005131-199206000-00022

[79] Ding L, He Z, Xiao H, Chai L, Xue F. Risk factors for postoperative wound complications of calcaneal fractures following plate fixation. Foot & Ankle International. 2013;**34**(9):1238-1244. DOI: 10.1177/1071100713484718

[80] Folk JW, Starr AJ, Early JS. Early wound complications of operative treatment of calcaneus fractures: Analysis of 190 fractures. Journal of Orthopaedic Trauma. 1999;**13**(5):369-372. DOI: 10.1097/00005131-199906000-00008

[81] Spierings KE, Min M, Nooijen LE, Swords MP, Schepers T. Managing the open calcaneal fracture: A systematic review. Foot and Ankle Surgery. 2019;**25**(6):707-713. DOI: 10.1016/j.fas.2018.10.005

[82] Cavadas PC, Landin L. Management of soft-tissue complications of the lateral approach for calcaneal fractures. Plastic and Reconstructive Surgery. 2007;**120**(2):459-466. DOI: 10.1097/01.prs.0000267418.66689.61

[83] Krishna D, Chaturvedi G, Khan MM, Cheruvu VPR, Laitonjam M, Minz R. Reconstruction of heel soft tissue defects: An algorithm based on our experience. World Journal of Plastic Surgery. 2021;**10**(3):63-72. DOI: 10.29252/wjps.10.3.63

[84] Yu X, Pang QJ, Chen L, Yang CC, Chen XJ. Postoperative complications after closed calcaneus fracture treated by open reduction and internal fixation: A review. The Journal of International Medical Research. 2014;**42**(1):17-25. DOI: 10.1177/0300060513495626

[85] Sanders R. Displaced intra-articular fractures of the calcaneus. The Journal of Bone and Joint Surgery. American Volume. 2000;**82**(2):225-250. DOI: 10.2106/00004623-200002000-00009

[86] Maskill JD, Bohay DR, Anderson JG. Calcaneus fractures: A review article. Foot and Ankle Clinics. 2005;**10**(3):463-489, vi. DOI: 10.1016/j.fcl.2005.03.002

[87] Reddy V, Fukuda T, Ptaszek AJ. Calcaneus malunion and nonunion. Foot and Ankle Clinics. 2007;**12**(1):125-135. DOI: 10.1016/j.fcl.2006.12.004

[88] Wang C, Huang D, Ma X, et al. Sustentacular screw placement with guidance during ORIF of calcaneal fracture: An anatomical specimen study. Journal of Orthopaedic Surgery and Research. 2017;**12**(1):78. DOI: 10.1186/s13018-017-0580-5